SPIRITUALITY IN PHARMACY PRACTICE

ACCLAIM FOR *SPIRITUALITY IN PHARMACY PRACTICE*

"Building on the well-established foundation of a biopsychosocial model of clinical practice, Nolen and colleagues offer a path for healthcare providers to add spiritual dimensions to the physical, emotional, and social considerations of a patient's well-being, fostering a truly holistic approach to care. By integrating empathy, active listening, and respect for diverse beliefs, the whole-person approach they suggest transforms treatment into meaningful connections that promote healing and trust."

Jonathan B. Perlin, MD, PhD, MSHA, MACP, FACMI, FAMIA
President and Chief Executive Officer
The Joint Commission enterprise

"We live in a time of tremendous turbulence throughout our culture, including healthcare. Advances in AI and other challenges cry out for the rediscovery of whole-person care that is patient focused. This wonderful book highlights the importance of attending to spirituality as a central component of whole-person care. Pharmacy is a front-line vocation where the opportunities for deep listening and engagement are prevalent, and this is a wise resource to spur deeper attentiveness."

L. Gregory Jones, PhD, MDiv
President
Belmont University

"The title of this critical contribution to patient-centered care could easily be changed to *Spirituality in Practice*, as the content's importance and applicability span the spectrum of healthcare providers. Importantly, while the book's focus is rightly on patients, it reminds us that by nourishing our patients' souls, we feed our own—a byproduct desperately needed in this time, when symptoms of burnout threaten the effectiveness of more than half of our healthcare colleagues."

Michael S. Woods, MD, MMM
Surgeon and Author

"*Spirituality in Pharmacy Practice* fills a void in the pharmacy literature by focusing on an often-ignored aspect of pharmaceutical care and pharmacy practice: the role of spirituality and faith in patient care. For many individuals, myself included, the role of faith is central to their identity and worldview. This book addresses the topic with thoughtfulness and care and should be an essential reading for all pharmacists."

Neil MacKinnon, PhD
President and Professor
Central Michigan University

SPIRITUALITY IN PHARMACY PRACTICE

Perspectives on Whole-Person Care

Agatha Nolen, PhD, MDiv, FASHP
Instructor
Duke University–Duke Divinity School
Durham, North Carolina

Marianne F. Ivey, PharmD, MPH, FASHP, FFIP
Professor Emerita, University of Cincinnati
Pharmacy Practice and Administrative Sciences
Seattle, Washington

Paul C. Walker, PharmD, FASHP, FMPA
Clinical Professor Emeritus of Pharmacy
University of Michigan College of Pharmacy
Belleville, Michigan

David A. Zilz, MS, FASHP, FPSW
Clinical Professor Emeritus of Pharmacy
University of Wisconsin Health and School of Pharmacy
Iola, Wisconsin

ashp®

Any correspondence regarding this publication should be sent to the publisher, American Society of Health-System Pharmacists, 4500 East-West Highway, Suite 900, Bethesda, MD 20814, attention: Special Publishing.

Senior Vice President, Professional Development and Publishing Office: Daniel J. Cobaugh, PharmD, DABAT, FAACT

Senior Editorial Director, Special Publishing: Ryan E. Owens, PharmD, BCPS

Editorial Coordinator, Special Publishing: Güneş Turhanlı, MA

Director, Production and Platform Services, Special Publishing: Johnna M. Hershey, BA

Production Services/Printing: Apex CoVantage, LLC/Sheridan

Cover Design: DeVall Advertising

Cover Art: Graph Rover - stock.adobe.com

Library of Congress Cataloging-in-Publication Data

A catalog record for this book is available from the Library of Congress.

The authorized representative in the EU for product safety and compliance is Mare Nostrum Group B.V., Mauritskade 21D, 1091 GC Amsterdam, The Netherlands; gpsr@mare-nostrum.co.uk

Print ISBN: 978-1-58528-771-0
PDF ISBN: 978-1-58528-772-7
ePub ISBN: 978-1-58528-773-4
DOI 10.37573/9781585287727

10 9 8 7 6 5 4 3 2 1

DEDICATION

To the pharmacists, student pharmacists, pharmacy technicians, and patients in all practice settings and of all religions or no religion, spiritual or not spiritual, who recognize that healing is not only of the body but is also influenced by values and beliefs. Your stories offer glimpses of pharmacy as a healing profession that encompasses not just medication expertise but presence and compassion in our interactions with patients, coworkers, and colleagues. We care for and about each other as whole persons, recognizing how our physical, mental, and spiritual needs contribute to our healthy well-being.

TABLE OF CONTENTS

Acknowledgments xiii
Preface xv
Editors/Contributors xvii
Introduction xxiii

A Voice Crying in the Wilderness 1
Daniel H. Albrant, PharmD, MDiv

More Than Reconciling Medications 5
Azadeh Ali-Moghaddam, PharmD

Loss of a Coworker: Bereavement in the Workplace 9
John A. Armitstead, MS, RPh, CPEL, FASHP

Spirituality and Pharmacy: A Collaborative Approach to Whole-Person Care 13
Rabia S. Atayee, PharmD, BCPS, APh, FAAHPM, FPPCP, and
Allison Kestenbaum, MA, MPA, BCC-PCHAC, ACPE Certified Educator

Vulnerability in Suffering 17
Angela Baalmann, PharmD, MS, BCACP

What About Forgiveness? A Reflection on the Spiritual Practice of Listening 21
Jake Blair, PharmD, CTHC

An Act of Compassion and Humanity for a Patient at the End of Life 25
Matthew D. Clark, PharmD

Love, Hope, Pharmacy, and Sisters 29
Melissa M. Corrigan, BS Pharm, CAE, FAPhA, FASHP

A Prescription for Hope 33
Kate Cozart, MEd, PharmD, BCPS, BCGP, BCACP

The Fate of Faith: Lessons from a Hospital Encounter 37
Jeremy Espeut, PharmD, MBA, MS

A Redirected Calling 41
Diane B. Ginsburg, PhD, MS, RPh, FASHP, DASPL

Holistic Pharmacist-Led Patient Care in a West African Hospital Setting 45
Anonymous

DOI: 10.37573/9781585287727.FM

The Power of Prayer 49
Elisa Greene, PharmD

Beyond the Guidelines: Practicing the Humanity of Medicine 53
Kevin Thomas Hatley, PharmD candidate

Establishing Patient Credibility in Long-Term Care Through Spirituality 55
Mark S. Johnson, PharmD, MACE, BCPS

A Call to Fill the Spiritual Gap in Holistic Care 59
Kendra A.N. Lucas, PharmD

Providence and Presence 63
James T. Miller, PharmD, BCCCP

Presence as Medicine: A Story of Unborn, Spirit, and Trust in Patient Care 67
Phuoc Anne Nguyen, PharmD, MS, BCPS, FTSHP

Amazing Grace 71
Agatha Nolen, PhD, MDiv, FASHP

A Whisper Before the Injection: A Lesson in Spiritual Presence 75
Alvena Noor, PharmD candidate

Honoring Faith in the Pharmacy Setting: Spiritual Encounters in Community Care 79
Sue Paul, RPh

The Healing Power of Prayer 83
Susan L. Ravnan, PharmD, FCSHP

***Cura Personalis* in the Dominican Republic** 87
Edward M. Saito, PharmD, BCACP, DPLA

A Pharmacist's Spiritual Journey While Working on American Indian Reservations 91
Kathryn Rose Thorsness Schultz, BS Pharm, PharmD, MPH, FASHP, FMSHP

Religious Education Meets Real-World Practice 95
Kathryn Schwaller, PharmD, MS

Role of Prayer in Managing Patients with HIV/AIDS 99
Gary H. Smith, PharmD, FASHP, FCCP, FAPhA

Celebrating Life After a Close Encounter with Death 103
Claudia N. Swenson, PharmD, FASHP

When Ripples Become Waves 107
Elva Angelique Van Devender, PhD, PharmD, BCPS, DPLA

My Traveling Companion 111
Carly B. Warner, PharmD, BCPS, BCGP

Self-Reflection Questions 115

ACKNOWLEDGMENTS

We acknowledge the following groups and individuals for their contributions to this book:

- The contributing authors and reviewers whose personal narratives bring our patients' spiritual needs to the forefront and provide evidence that caring and presence happen in all practice settings and involve caregivers and patients of all religions and spirituality.
- Our patients who inspire us with their resilience, tenacity, and endurance in striving for healthy well-being.
- The Special Publishing staff at ASHP—especially Ryan Owens and Güneş Turhanlı—for their patience, encouragement, and assistance throughout the process.
- Our nonpharmacy friends who have provided advice and enthusiasm for the book's concept and shared their own stories of their healthcare journeys and how religion and spirituality have impacted their care.

Agatha Nolen, Marianne F. Ivey, Paul C. Walker, David A. Zilz

To Margaret Jane Dodson, my nurse friend, who taught me that caring for a patient's spiritual needs is often a spontaneous action of listening and caring, which can occur in any healthcare setting; and to her father, Seawell Brandau, who always reminds me that the patient is at the center of the experience, and patients play an active role by starting the conversation with their healthcare provider about their spiritual needs.

Agatha Nolen, PhD, MDiv, FASHP

To my editor/colleagues of this book: To Dave, a long-admired mentor, colleague, and friend and our conversations on spirituality that led to published articles and eventually this book; to Agatha, whose strong spiritual presence I've witnessed since we served on the ASHP Board of Directors together and whose writing and information-handling skills were central to the book's completion; and to Paul, whose ASHP inaugural address was evidence that he had a spiritual strength above and beyond his expertise in pharmacy, therapeutics, and teaching. Much gratitude to my dear family, lifelong friends, colleagues, and patients who taught me about grace; the desire to live a meaningful, value-anchored life; and the power of prayer.

Marianne F. Ivey, PharmD, MPH, FASHP, FFIP

To my wife, Kathy, who lives with amazing grace, and to the pastors who taught me what it means to live out my faith in the everyday work of my hands with integrity and compassion. The example of your lives helped shape how I approach my professional calling—as a pharmacist, educator, and Christian minister. From you, I learned that faith and excellence in practice can walk hand in hand, that caring for patients is more than clinical work—it's whole-person ministry—and that nurturing and teaching health professions' students is a sacred trust.

Paul C. Walker, PharmD, FASHP, FMPA

DOI: 10.37573/9781585287727.FM

To my co-editors: What a wonderful experience at this stage of my life to participate with such a very talented, dedicated, and knowledgeable team of individuals in developing this book. The effort and contribution of each of you during the entire process has been an inspiration to me. To all the authors: I appreciate how you tell compelling stories of your experiences in assessing the variety of needs that you encountered and how you responded to those needs with compassion and grace. You are all to be commended. To my family, especially in memory of my wife, MaryAnn, who passed away during this effort: This represents our journey in faith together. My wife would have been delighted and smiled with approval for all these stories. The foundation of her life was spiritual growth. To my daughter, Kristin, and granddaughters: You are all encouragement to me as I see you growing in your understanding and wisdom.

David A. Zilz, MS, FASHP, FPSW

PREFACE

Whole-person care is an integrative approach that acknowledges the interconnection of body, mind, and spirit in health and healing. Increasingly, across healthcare, there is growing awareness that when we care for the whole person—listening to their story, respecting their values, and addressing emotional and spiritual needs—patients experience better clinical outcomes and providers find greater meaning in their work. This holistic perspective is reshaping clinical education, practice, and policy by encouraging providers to address the full spectrum of patient needs for sustained healing and wellness.

Does this shift toward whole-person care have significant implications for our role as pharmacists, student pharmacists, and pharmacy technicians? As we fulfill our responsibilities to help patients manage their medications to achieve optimal physical and mental well-being, we may be tempted to neglect religion and spirituality as components of whole-person care. Because of time constraints, timidity, fear, or "political correctness," we may avoid having meaningful conversations with our patients about their spiritual needs.

As we talked with our pharmacy colleagues and patients, we were encouraged to look more deeply at what whole-person means for pharmaceutical care and how this perspective can transform both our practice and our relationships with those we serve. We reviewed the significant body of literature that demonstrates the value of addressing spiritual needs and its mostly positive impact on health-related outcomes in heart disease, hypertension, cerebrovascular disease, and cancer. Greater religious or spiritual involvement has been shown to predict a significant reduction in mortality in the majority of studies. Integrating religion and spirituality into the care that we provide can improve health behaviors, such as cigarette smoking cessation, exercise, and diet.

As we worked through our literature review, we felt that something was largely absent: the personal stories from colleagues showing how attending to patients' spiritual needs affected both patients and providers. This book, *Spirituality in Pharmacy Practice: Perspectives on Whole-Person Care*, aims to fill that gap and provide practical examples of how providers and patients communicate about spiritual needs. We hope that many groups will find value in this compilation of 29 unique stories. We anticipate that schools and colleges of pharmacy and other healthcare-focused schools will incorporate this book into their curricula in ethics courses or as a broader curriculum on whole-person care. We envision that senior citizen groups, religious groups, and other nonclinicians might use this in a book club format where a few stories are read and discussed. Most of all, we hope that practitioners and patients will see themselves in these stories and be comfortable starting a conversation about religion and spirituality in their healthcare encounters.

Each chapter is a unique story. The book is ordered by the contributing author's last name. In cases where a patient is named, a pseudonym is used to protect privacy. There are stories from pharmacists and student pharmacists practicing in the United States and internationally. They involve practitioners and patients from many different religions and practice settings; often, the religious preferences of the provider and patient are not the same.

DOI: 10.37573/9781585287727.FM

Our hope is that you will find yourself in at least one of these stories and be encouraged to examine the impact that religion and spirituality have on your well-being as we travel on our healthcare journeys together.

Agatha Nolen, PhD, MDiv, FASHP
Marianne F. Ivey, PharmD, MPH, FASHP, FFIP
Paul C. Walker, PharmD, FASHP, FMPA
David A. Zilz, MS, FASHP, FPSW

Editors

Editors

Agatha Nolen, PhD, MDiv, FASHP

Instructor
Duke University–Duke Divinity School
Durham, North Carolina

Marianne F. Ivey, PharmD, MPH, FASHP, FFIP

Professor Emerita, University of Cincinnati
Pharmacy Practice and Administrative Sciences
Seattle, Washington

Paul C. Walker, PharmD, FASHP, FMPA

Clinical Professor Emeritus of Pharmacy
University of Michigan College of Pharmacy
Belleville, Michigan

David A. Zilz, MS, FASHP, FPSW

Clinical Professor Emeritus of Pharmacy
University of Wisconsin Health and School of Pharmacy
Iola, Wisconsin

Contributors

Daniel H. Albrant, PharmD, MDiv

Pastor
Mineral–Mount Pleasant United Methodist Charge
Mineral, Virginia

Azadeh Ali-Moghaddam, PharmD

Clinical Pharmacy Lecturer III
College of Pharmacy
University of Michigan
Ann Arbor, Michigan

John A. Armitstead, MS, RPh, CPEL, FASHP

Vice President, Pharmacy Services
Lee Health Pharmacy
Fort Myers, Florida

DOI: 10.37573/9781585287727.FM

Rabia S. Atayee, PharmD, BCPS, APh, FAAHPM, FPPCP
Professor of Clinical Pharmacy
Associate Dean
SSPPS Office of Admissions and Recruitment (SOAR)
Palliative Care Specialist
Founding Member
Society of Pain & Palliative Care Pharmacists
Center for Compassionate Communication, Affiliate Faculty
La Jolla, California

Angela Baalmann, PharmD, MS, BCACP
Fred Wilson School of Pharmacy
High Point University
High Point, North Carolina

Jake Blair, PharmD, CTHC
Senior Clinical Pharmacist
Blue Cross North Carolina
Durham, North Carolina
Affiliated Faculty
Harding University College of Pharmacy
Searcy, Arkansas
Adjunct Professor
Campbell University College of Pharmacy & Health Sciences
Buies Creek, North Carolina

Matthew D. Clark, PharmD
Clinical Pharmacy Specialist
The University of Texas MD Anderson Cancer Center
Houston, Texas

Melissa M. Corrigan, BS Pharm, CAE, FAPhA, FASHP
Adjunct Assistant Professor, Department of Pharmacy Practice
University of Iowa, College of Pharmacy
Creator & Host, MelisRxScripts Podcast
Iowa City, Iowa

Kate Cozart, MEd, PharmD, BCPS, BCGP, BCACP
Clinical Pharmacist Practitioner, Primary Care
Veterans Affairs Tennessee Valley Healthcare System
Clarksville, Tennessee

Jeremy Espeut, PharmD, MBA, MS

Acute Care Pharmacy Operations
Baptist Health South Florida
Miami, Florida

Diane B. Ginsburg, PhD, MS, RPh, FASHP, DASPL

Clinical Professor, Pharmacy Practice Division
Associate Dean for Healthcare Partnerships
G.D. Searle Endowed Fellow in Pharmacy
Provost's Distinguished Leadership & Service Professor
The University of Texas at Austin
College of Pharmacy
Austin, Texas

Elisa Greene, PharmD

Professor of Pharmacy Practice
Belmont University
Clinical Pharmacist
Siloam Health
Nashville, Tennessee

Kevin Thomas Hatley, PharmD candidate

Thomas J. Long School of Pharmacy
University of the Pacific
Stockton, California

Mark S. Johnson, PharmD, MACE, BCPS

Professor of Pharmacy Practice
Bernard J. Dunn School of Pharmacy
Shenandoah University
Winchester, Virginia

Allison Kestenbaum, MA, MPA, BCC-PCHAC, ACPE Certified Educator

Manager of Spiritual Care & Clinical Pastoral Education
UC San Diego Health
Associate Clinical Professor, Department of Medicine, Department of Geriatrics and Palliative Care
UC San Diego Health Sciences
San Diego, California

Kendra A.N. Lucas, PharmD

Director of Clinical Services (Fmr.)
Hope Healthcare Services
Avon, Indiana

James T. Miller, PharmD, BCCCP

Clinical Pharmacy Specialist—Surgical Critical Care
Adjunct Clinical Assistant Professor
Residency Program Director—PGY2 Critical Care Pharmacy
University of Michigan Health
University of Michigan College of Pharmacy
University of Michigan
Ann Arbor, Michigan

Phuoc Anne Nguyen, PharmD, MS, BCPS, FTSHP

Specialty Pharmacy Operations Manager
Vital Care of Houston Specialty Pharmacy
Richmond, Texas

Alvena Noor, PharmD candidate

Ziauddin University
Karachi, Sindh, Pakistan

Sue Paul, RPh

Founder
SyneRxgy Consulting LLC
Co-Founder
PGx101, LLC
Clinical Pharmacist
Crossroad Health Center and NeighborHub Health
Cincinnati, Ohio

Susan L. Ravnan, PharmD, FCSHP

Professor Emerita
Department of Pharmacy Practice
Thomas J. Long School of Pharmacy
University of the Pacific
Stockton, California

Edward M. Saito, PharmD, BCACP, DPLA

Associate Professor
Pacific University School of Pharmacy
Hillsboro, Oregon

Kathryn Rose Thorsness Schultz, BS Pharm, PharmD, MPH, FASHP, FMSHP

Staff Pharmacist
Quentin N. Burdick Memorial Health Care Facility
Turtle Mountain Reservation
Belcourt, North Dakota

Kathryn Schwaller, PharmD, MS

Pharmacy Operations Coordinator
Cincinnati, Ohio

Gary H. Smith, PharmD, FASHP, FCCP, FAPhA

Clinical Professor
University of Arizona College of Pharmacy
Tucson, Arizona

Claudia N. Swenson, PharmD

Clinical Coordinator (Ret.)
Confluence Hospital
Wenatchee, Washington

Elva Angelique Van Devender, PhD, PharmD, BCPS, DPLA

Clinical Pharmacy Supervisor Medication Assistance Program
Providence St. Joseph Health—Providence Medical Group, Oregon Region
Portland, Oregon

Carly B. Warner, PharmD, BCPS, BCGP

Shepherd Center
Atlanta, Georgia
UNC Health Rex at Holly Springs
Holly Springs, North Carolina

INTRODUCTION

Pharmacists are important members of the healthcare team and, as healthcare providers, commit themselves to "consider the welfare of humanity and relief of suffering as primary concerns."[1] As human beings, patients are not just made up of isolated body parts that need periodic mending like a machine, but instead they are living, breathing organisms with individual needs who require attention to optimize their best life. In addition to physical and mental health needs, many patients claim a religious or spiritual component that also impacts their overall health. In caring for the welfare of humanity, healthcare providers should address the whole mind-body-spirit triad.

Many definitions of "religion" and "spirituality" appear in research studies and on social media. Throughout this book, we have utilized common definitions used in clinical practice where "religion" is a system of beliefs and practices that unite adherents into a community with a shared vision for attaining union with, or the experience of, the divine or transcendent. In contrast, "spirituality" is defined by the patient themselves but broadly encompasses a set of beliefs, practices, and ways of being that are intended to assist in attaining union with, or experience of, the divine or transcendent. These definitions are similar but differ in where the emphasis is placed: religion pertains to a community, whereas spirituality pertains to the individual.[2] As spirituality is defined by each patient, it is important that healthcare providers practice presence—intentionally focusing awareness, attention, and empathy on the patient in order to fully connect, understand, and support them—with close listening in dialogue and engagement with their patients.[2]

Researchers have found that the effects of spiritual and religious beliefs/practices have significant impacts on health. Spiritual and religious beliefs may influence medical decision-making and adherence with treatment regimens. Koenig et al. concluded that healthcare professionals should be willing to discuss religious and spiritual matters with patients rather than ignoring or avoiding them. Two factors should encourage these discussions: (1) religious and spiritual beliefs are widespread among patients and often influence how they cope with mental or physical illness; and (2) when we address these spiritual needs, well-being, healthcare outcomes, and quality of life can be improved.[2]

Supporting these patient needs may be as simple as verbal recognition of the patient's expressed spirituality or may involve simple interventions (eg, providing accommodations that enable the patient to practice their religion; praying with the patient if requested; providing a referral to pastoral care, such as chaplains or community-based clerics) to address spiritual needs.[2] For patients who are not religious or spiritual, Siegel et al. recommend a state-of-the art secular medical model "to cure sometimes, to relieve often, to comfort always."[3]

What does this look like for healthcare providers and patients in day-to-day clinical practice? How do pharmacists, student pharmacists, and pharmacy technicians engage in this kind of care?

Some pharmacy schools may offer training in ethical decision-making, but few offer practical advice on incorporating spiritual care into everyday practice. Pharmacists are not specially trained in meeting spiritual needs like chaplains or clerics, but as one human being

DOI: 10.37573/9781585287727.FM

who cares about another, we can acknowledge the spiritual dimension of our patients. As you will see in the 29 narratives in this book, pharmacists, student pharmacists, and pharmacy technicians can engage their patients in conversations about spiritual needs that are patient-centered without proselytizing or coercion. Patients should also feel free to start the conversation about any spiritual needs that may impact their care.

For example, in the hospital setting, upon admission, most patients are asked if they have a religious preference. Acknowledging their response as documented in the medical record may be the first step to a larger conversation. "Mr. Jones, I see that you responded in your admission history that you are Jewish. Is there someone at your synagogue who you'd like me to contact to let them know that you are here?" The answer may be "yes," or it may be "no," but now a bridge has been created to an open conversation that the patient may choose to pursue. When you walk into a patient's room, you may notice on their bedside a Bible, a rosary, or prayer beads, such as a "mala" used in Hinduism, Buddhism, Jainism, and Sikhism; "misbaha" used in Islam and some Judaic traditions; Anglican prayer beads; or Baha'i prayer beads used in the Baha'i faith. These observations may also serve as conversation-starters. "I noticed your Bible. Are you studying something specific?" "What beautiful prayer beads. Do you pray with them every day?" As a healthcare provider, you are merely acknowledging that religion/spirituality is important to your patient.

What if the admission history says, "no religious preference" or "atheist" or "agnostic"? Confirming the patient's response acknowledges that you care about the patient enough to ask even when no spiritual views or needs are voiced.

Healthcare providers should be willing to have a conversation with every patient to identify whether they have any spiritual needs alongside any physical and mental health concerns. Pharmacists, student pharmacists, and pharmacy technicians may not be trained experts in meeting religious or spiritual needs, but as these narratives show, we can provide conversation and comfort. We care about providing optimal health outcomes, but we also care about our patients (and their families) as human beings. Our goal is their goal: ultimately to flourish in all dimensions of their lives. Pharmacists are beginning to document their understanding of the importance of spirituality in the healing process, particularly in critical illness and end-of-life care.[4-6] This publication will share experiences of pharmacist-provided spiritual care.

We acknowledge our contributing authors who have shared personal encounters that have been meaningful to their patients and themselves. We hope that as a healthcare provider or as a patient, you will see yourself in at least one of these stories and be willing to have a conversation about spirituality at your next provider–patient encounter.

References

1. American Pharmacists Association. https://www.pharmacist.com/About/Oath-of-a-Pharmacist. Accessed March 14, 2026.
2. Koenig HG, Vanderweele TJ, Peteet JR. *Handbook of Religion and Health.* 3rd ed. Oxford University Press; 2024.
3. Siegel MD. "To comfort always." *Yale School of Medicine News.* June 24, 2018. https://medicine.yale.edu/news-article/to-comfort-always. Accessed March 14, 2026.

4. Ivey MF, Vest TA, Zilz DA. The need for increased education and training of pharmacy learners in the care of older, critically ill, and end-of-life patients. *Am J Health-Syst Pharm.* 2021;78(14):1336-1340. https://doi.org/10.1093/ajhp/zxab177
5. Nolen AL, Ivey MF, Walker PC. Spiritual practices and beliefs as a social determinant of health: when will the profession of pharmacy address the whole body-mind-spirit triad? *Am J Health-Syst Pharm.* 2023;80(16):1101-1105. https://doi.org/10.1093/ajhp/zxad081
6. Zilz DA. When difficult conversations occur, will you be ready? *Am J Health-Syst Pharm.* 2021;78(17):1600-1602. https://doi.org/10.1093/ajhp/zxab213

A Voice Crying in the Wilderness

Daniel H. Albrant
PharmD, MDiv

I began my clinical practice in intensive care units (ICUs) in a mid-sized hospital in 1989. Clinical pharmacists in this practice environment were uncommon in those days, especially outside of large academic medical centers. Critical care pharmacists frequently engage in life-and-death situations. This was especially the case 35 years ago when approximately one-third of all ICU admissions would die before leaving the hospital. The ICU is a high-tech, low-touch environment, where it is easy to lose sight of the humanity of the person in the bed. They tend to become a constellation of symptoms and brokenness that require intervention and curing. Working in such an environment requires that practitioners develop thick skins or that they armor up before beginning their shift, preparing themselves psychologically, emotionally, and sometimes spiritually to face the anticipated stress of their work.

Ten years into my critical care practice, I began to burn out. The intensity of the work coupled with the suffering and death of patients became a burden that grew heavier by the day. Some medical providers continued to hold that death was a failure, which added stress to me personally as well as to my team. I needed a perspective on life and death that could help me let go of this burden so that I could continue to practice in the place to which I believed I was uniquely gifted and called to care. I needed a way to put death into perspective—not as a failure, but as a normal part of human life. After all, life has a 100% mortality rate; none of us will get out alive.

As I wrestled with how to move forward in my professional life, my home church began a Stephen Ministry program. Stephen Ministry is a Christian caregiving ministry that equips trained laypeople in a congregation to provide confidential, one-to-one, Christ-centered care to people who are experiencing difficulties in life. It uses tools, such as active listening, nonjudgmental presence, weekly meetings, healthy boundary setting, and group assessment of the relationship. It teaches dependence on God for guidance through prayer. I became a Stephen Minister and eventually, a Stephen Leader. Leadership required intentional spiritual development, which taught me personal spiritual disciplines, such as contemplation and many forms of prayer. Interestingly, it brought me into a deep and abiding relationship with a chaplain at my hospital.

DOI: 10.37573/9781585287727.001

My relationship with the hospital chaplain, which was new for me, helped me to discuss spiritual matters in the workplace. Suddenly, I realized that I was not alone in my struggle to live out my spirituality in the workplace. I was not just "a voice crying out in the wilderness" by myself; there were others who sensed a need to change their perspective on life.

The chaplain and I met once a week before patient rounds to share a cup of coffee and our lives. We would chat about the lack of attention to the spiritual needs of patients and families and how we might address those issues. Those weekly conversations eventually led us to develop an approach to help ICU professionals speak about the burdens they carried because of their work. We conversed with nurses and physicians about how they were feeling, about the suffering and death they faced, and how this burden was impacting them. We tried to do this during work hours but found that few people would engage in the discussion. People were reticent during work to let down their guard or to take off the armor around their emotions. How could they function if they left themselves vulnerable to the emotions that were their constant companion throughout their day? They felt they could only do their lifesaving work if they kept a certain emotional distance from it.

The chaplain and I were disappointed that our initiative was not as effective as planned; however, it changed my interaction with the staff. I began to have more one-on-one conversations with nurses, physicians, and other staff caring for the patients in the ICUs. In these conversations, they described how their own spirituality helped them to infuse the environment with a deeper sense of humanity. They began inviting me to participate in family meetings to contribute my pharmaceutical knowledge, clinical expertise, and spiritual perspective to the discussions.

In time, I set aside my ICU pharmacy practice to pursue seminary training and follow my calling as a church pastor. During seminary, I served as an on-call hospital chaplain, which provided me the first opportunity to document in a medical record my spiritual assessment of a patient and their spiritual needs. I met with people in crisis: in emergency departments after accidents, grieving the death of a loved one, when facing decisions about removing life support, or coping with a new and tragic diagnosis.

Through my chaplaincy, I became involved in teaching and mentoring medical students. Their medical school curriculum included a professional development program that paired physicians with experts in the social and psychological sciences. I was chosen by the medical school to participate in the program because of my clinical experience and spiritual training. This opportunity allowed me to mentor students throughout their 4 years of study, encouraging them to nurture their compassionate, human side. I guided them to pay close attention to the daily lives of their patients—understanding not only medical issues, but also the struggles, concerns, and challenges that shape each individual's experience. By fostering empathy and genuine curiosity, I helped students to recognize the importance of caring for patients as whole people, not just as medical cases. These young people were from a variety of spiritual backgrounds; some had no defined faith at all. However, through patient vignettes with trained actors, we gave them experience in navigating challenging patient conversations.

Although I was the only religious professional among the nonphysicians, my voice was valued by colleagues and by the students. Being able to bring my perspective—as a clinician and as a spiritual person—was helpful to students and medical colleagues as they wrestled with the "slings and arrows of outrageous fortune" that characterizes many of our lives.

Over the past 38 years, I have observed the increasing integration of spirituality into patient care, recognizing it as a crucial factor influencing health outcomes. Professional chaplains are much more common now than they ever were, and I encourage all pharmacists to engage them in conversation. No matter what your spirituality may be, these ecumenical spiritual professionals can open your heart and mind to discover how to use the fullness of yourself in your practice. None of us needs to be a lonesome voice crying out in the wilderness; we are surrounded by spiritual people living very human lives.

More Than Reconciling Medications

Azadeh Ali-Moghaddam
PharmD

It was the last day of my inpatient advanced pharmacy practice rotation. Like every other morning, I walked through the halls with my list of patients, prepared to complete one of my routine responsibilities: medication reconciliation. It's a deceptively simple phrase—"med rec"—but one of the most critical steps in safe patient care. It involves gathering a patient's complete home medication history and carefully comparing it against their inpatient therapies. Done well, it prevents omissions, duplications, and dangerous errors. Done poorly, it can mean harm.

That morning, I had already worked through most of my list when I reached my final patient. Her case looked like the perfect way to end the day: simple. Her home medication list contained only one item, a multivitamin. Compared with the complex, multipage inpatient list in her chart, the contrast was stark.

"This one should be quick," I thought, imagining myself finishing the rotation strong. However, as I approached her room, I noticed an unusual handwritten sign taped to her door: **Do not enter before you are allowed in!**

I paused. I had seen "Isolation" or "Neutropenic Precautions" signs before, but never something like this. I knocked softly and waited.

After a long moment, I heard a faint, hesitant voice: "Come in."

When I stepped inside, the reason for the sign became immediately clear. The patient—a young woman—was curled under her bedsheets, awkwardly covering her bald head. The air felt heavy with sadness. Her eyes were swollen; her face streaked from tears. She didn't look at me directly, only glanced briefly, making sure to hide her head beneath the covers.

I gently introduced myself. "I'm a pharmacy student here to talk about your medications, if you feel up for it."

She gave a small shrug, expressionless, as though nothing mattered anymore.

I glanced at her record. "I only see a multivitamin on your home list. Is that accurate?"

At once, her composure broke. She burst into tears, her sobs filling the room.

"Yes," she managed to say between breaths. "That is accurate. I was healthy. I took care of myself—I ate well, exercised, never smoked, never even around

DOI: 10.37573/9781585287727.002

secondhand smoke. I took my multivitamin every day. I cared for my family. I did everything right."

Her voice shook as frustration blended with despair.

"Then I caught a cold. Just a simple cold. I started coughing, and it lasted for weeks. My doctor thought it might be an infection, so he prescribed antibiotics. They didn't help, so he gave me a stronger course. Still nothing. Finally, they sent me for some tests to check for a stubborn lung infection."

She stopped, covering her face with trembling hands.

"That's when they found it. Stage 4 lung cancer. Six months to live."

Tears poured down her cheeks, and I felt my own tears welling up in response. She pulled the blanket higher over her bald scalp, as though hiding could protect her from the reality pressing in.

"I have four children," she cried. "My youngest is only 6 months old. I'm 34. I don't want to die. I have so many hopes and dreams. I just want to see my baby walk."

The rawness of her grief hit me with a force I hadn't experienced before. In that moment, her pain filled the entire room.

She went on to describe how another hospital employee had visited her earlier in the week, telling her to repent and accept her destiny. "I didn't like the interaction," she admitted softly. "I didn't feel heard. It all just feels so unfair."

I hesitated, unsure what to say. This was not something my pharmacy textbooks had prepared me for. Yet silence felt wrong.

"May I sit beside you?" I asked.

She nodded slightly.

Sitting on the bed beside her, I said quietly, "I'm so sorry for everything you are going through. I honestly don't have the right words. But if you are open to it, I'd like to offer two things."

She looked toward me, curious despite her grief.

"First," I said, "while no one has a guaranteed tomorrow, I believe in God and in His miracles. I have a close group of friends who are believers, too. If you'd like, I can ask them to pray for you."

Her face changed, a tiny spark of hope breaking through her tears. "Oh, please. ANYTHING that could help. Please do."

"I will," I promised.

"Second," I added, "I can show you how to cover your head beautifully—so you don't have to hide under blankets. Would you like that?"

For the first time since I entered the room, she gave a real smile—small but genuine. She nodded.

I explained that I was a practicing Muslim and wore a scarf daily. I loosened my own scarf and demonstrated different styles: how to tie a bow at the side, how to drape it so it resembled hair, how to add elegance with the simplest adjustments. Her eyes followed each movement closely, and her expression softened with every example.

Then, I pulled up a website selling seamless silk turbans designed for cancer patients—soft, stylish, and gentle on sensitive skin.

Her tears returned, but they were no longer only tears of grief. Gratitude shone through.

"Thank you," she whispered. "Thank you for giving me hope. For giving me something positive. For seeing me—not just my illness."

What I had expected to be a routine 5-minute medication reconciliation stretched into a 1½ hour conversation. We spoke not only about medications, but about life—her children, her dreams, her fears, and her faith. We laughed through tears. The hospital room, heavy with sorrow when I entered, felt lighter by the time I left.

By the end of our conversation, her shoulders had eased. Her voice carried less weight. Even if only for a brief moment, she seemed at peace.

That was my last patient on my last day of rotation. I never saw her again, nor did I learn what became of her. But she has never left me.

Pharmacy training emphasizes knowledge, precision, and safety. But this encounter showed me something greater: patients are never just their diagnoses. Behind every chart is a human being with a story, with dreams, with a future that they are desperate to hold onto.

That day taught me that the most powerful interventions aren't always clinical. Sometimes, they are human. A kind word. A prayer. Even a scarf tied with dignity.

Empathy is not about fixing someone's suffering. It's about entering into it, even briefly, and helping them feel less alone. Hope, fragile as it is, matters. It may not cure disease, but it heals something inside.

I often think about that 34-year-old mother. Did she live long enough to see her baby's first steps? Did she hear her child laugh and call her name? I will never know. But I choose to believe she did—that she received moments of joy that medicine alone could not promise. Her memory remains a compass in my career. It reminds me that pharmacy is not only about medications, but about people. It is about showing up fully present in moments of vulnerability.

That last day on rotation taught me more than any lecture or guideline. It taught me that the heart of healthcare is, and always will be, human connection.

I carry with me the hope that somewhere, somehow, she saw her baby walk.

Loss of a Coworker: Bereavement in the Workplace

John A. Armitstead
MS, RPh, CPEL, FASHP

Yesterday morning began like any other, with the team ready to face another busy day in our community pharmacy. But the ordinary rhythm of the day shifted abruptly when Lacey (not her real name), who was always on time and rarely missed a shift, had not yet arrived. What began as a moment of quiet concern became something far more heartbreaking—a sudden and unexpected loss of one of our own. When we called to check on her status according to our schedule, a family member who answered her mobile phone informed us that Lacey had passed away overnight. As a single mother, it was her young child who was first to make the traumatic and shocking discovery.

In that moment of discovery, nothing in our pharmacy mattered as much as the people who stood beside us in our daily practice. We lost not only a coworker; we lost a friend, trusted colleague, and part of the fabric of our shared workplace. The grief in the pharmacy was immediate, unexpected, and palpable. Behind every individual, in every role and responsibility, is a human being who touches the lives of others in ways big and small. We are all interconnected.

In the fast-paced, professional, and technical world of pharmacy, it can be easy to focus solely on prescriptions, protocols, and clinical outcomes. But at the heart of this profession lies compassion, empathy, and human connection, and we are rooted in these values. I have heard often that many of us entered into the profession of pharmacy simply to help people.

Spirituality in pharmacy is not limited to religious belief but rather extends to recognizing the dignity, worth, and shared humanity of every person who crosses our path. It invites us to offer more than medication and care delivery; it invites us to offer presence, kindness, and care in moments of vulnerability and need.

In this spirit, I reflect on the recent loss of a cherished coworker, whose passing left an undeniable void in our workplace and in our hearts. They were a member of our health-system pharmacy team that is bound together by our commitment to the betterment of the lives of others. As we managed ourselves during the stages of grief—of denial, anger and dismay, bargaining, sadness and depression, and acceptance—we needed each other more acutely than we perceived on a daily basis. The grief that followed the death of a colleague is a profound reminder of the bonds we share beyond the professional roles that we occupy. As we accepted this loss, we

DOI: 10.37573/9781585287727.003

honored their memory by holding close the values of compassion and connection that defined their presence among us.

I have served in the profession of pharmacy for nearly 50 years, most recently as Vice President for Pharmacy Services in a large health system and have experienced the death of a colleague many times. It is never the same; the response and reactions vary based on the person, the team, and family circumstances. As a health-system pharmacy leader, I have learned that when a team member dies suddenly, a leader must respond to the team's needs with empathy, care, and clarity as they face the loss. It may also be a time to allow others to lead and for individual or group expressions of grief. Here are potential actions to consider:

Immediate Response

- Acknowledge the loss: Inform the team promptly with sensitivity. Avoid speculation about the cause of death.
- Contact human resources: Ensure proper procedures and notifications are followed.
- Support the family: Express condolences and offer support and contact numbers, facilitating employee benefits or employee assistance programs.

Supporting the Team

- Provide space for grief: Allow employees time to process the loss. Some may need temporary or more prolonged time off or counseling support. Remember that some employees may be closer and more deeply impacted than others. Allow for individual or group periods of work cessation.
- Hold impromptu or scheduled meetings: Create a safe space for the team to share thoughts, memories, and emotions.
- Offer resources: Provide access to spiritual services if available, Employee Assistance Programs (EAPs), or grief counseling services.

Managing Work Responsibilities

- Assess workload redistribution: Avoid overwhelming remaining team members; consider temporary support. Focus on urgent and important tasks, allowing delays on tasks that can be accomplished later.
- Adjust deadlines if possible: Recognize the emotional impact and allow flexibility where needed.
- Honor their contributions: Acknowledge the employee's work and legacy in a meaningful way.

Long-Term Considerations

- Memorialize thoughtfully: Consider a tribute, such as a moment of silence, donation, or a memory book. Perhaps your organization has a memorial garden or other method of commemorating the loss of an employee (flowers, trees, stepping stone, plaque).

- Monitor team morale: Check in regularly with staff to ensure ongoing emotional well-being.
- Reflect and improve policies or actions: Review how the organization handles such events and refine support systems, if needed.

Is a prayer appropriate in the workplace? I personally believe it is. Perhaps an interfaith prayer or reflection is best, one that focuses on the person, the connection to the team, and the realization that family is vitally important to the person's immediate circle. For example:

> *"We pause in this moment to honor the life of our colleague and friend, whose presence we will deeply miss.*
>
> *We are grateful for the time we shared, for the kindness, dedication, and spirit which they brought into our lives and our workplace.*
>
> *In this time of sorrow, we may find comfort in one another. May peace surround their loved ones and may strength and healing guide us all through this loss.*
>
> *Let us remember our dear colleague with gratitude and carry forward the good they left behind.*
>
> *May we find moments of stillness to reflect, to grieve, and to hope.*
>
> *With compassion in our hearts, we lift this prayer."*

Loss of a colleague is a very challenging time for a pharmacy leader. My greatest advice would be to take the time necessary for expressions of impact for your colleagues and attempt to make a connection with the family. This is not the time for avoidance and inconsequential actions. We should not allow ourselves to be possessed by inaction. It is a time for recognition, impact, reflection, and response. It is a time to truly exhibit the community spirit and interconnectedness of us all.

On a personal level, I would like to close this essay with a reflection that in moments of sorrow, I am reminded of the promise in Isaiah 40:31: *"But those who hope in the Lord will renew in strength; they will soar on wings like eagles, they will run and not grow weary, they will walk and not be faint."* As we honor Lacey's life and grieve her passing, may this truth bring us comfort and assurance. In time, may our hearts be lifted, our spirits renewed, and our strength restored through hope and faith.

Spirituality and Pharmacy: A Collaborative Approach to Whole-Person Care

Rabia S. Atayee
PharmD, BCPS, APh, FAAHPM, FPPCP

Allison Kestenbaum
MA, MPA, BCC-PCHAC, ACPE Certified Educator

As pharmacists, it is essential to recognize that we care for whole people, not just physical conditions. The whole-person care approach acknowledges that various dimensions, including physical, psychosocial, practical, social, and spiritual domains, can all influence a patient's health behaviors, including medication adherence and overall treatment outcomes.[1] Practical challenges, such as being unable to afford a medication or not understanding how to take it properly, can directly affect whether the patient uses it as prescribed, ultimately impacting its effectiveness. Similarly, a patient's spiritual beliefs may shape their healthcare decisions, such as preferences for certain treatments or use of alternative therapies, or their perspectives on illness and healing.

I (Atayee) have been a palliative care pharmacist for 19 years. I am originally from Afghanistan, and my family and I are practicing Muslims. In my years of practice, I have had the privilege of providing care to patients from a wide range of spiritual and religious backgrounds, many of whom hold beliefs different from my own. Yet, that has never prevented me from recognizing the importance of spirituality in their care or from supporting their spiritual needs with respect.

Understanding and assessing a patient's spiritual needs as part of routine care can help pharmacists build stronger therapeutic relationships and provide more personalized, respectful, and effective care. In palliative care, this work is best done in true collaboration with a chaplain, whose perspective is essential to optimizing care and health outcomes.

Palliative care is interprofessional care for serious illness that treats the whole person. The bio-psycho-social-spiritual approach in palliative care makes it so that chaplains have always been considered one of the "core disciplines" on the team, working literally side by side with pharmacists, social workers, physicians, and nurses.[2] The chaplain's job is to assess spiritual distress and spiritual needs (including resources) of all patients and their loved ones—whether they are of the same

DOI: 10.37573/9781585287727.004

faith background as me, a different one, or do not affiliate in any particular way. This sometimes surprises others; how can I (Kestenbaum) provide spiritual care to someone who is not from the same faith tradition? How can I provide spiritual care to someone who is not religious? Chaplains aim to be curious and humble and work to create space for those in our care, so they can express their values and what is most important to them in their medical treatment.

As a palliative care pharmacist, I (Atayee) am grateful to have a strong spiritual practice and connection on which I can draw for personal strength and fortitude in my daily work. I also find inspiration through my faith, which values interconnection, mystery, and the wonderful diversity of ways in which humans relate to that which is greater than any one of us. Even if a patient discloses their faith or cultural background to me, this only tells me a small part of their story. I collaborate with the interprofessional team to identify what gives the patient meaning, connection, and peace, and then help guide the team in integrating these values into their care.

I (Atayee) recall visiting a patient with metastatic breast cancer with one of my physician colleagues. The patient shared that prayer brought her hope and comfort. She identified as Christian and asked us to pray with her. We held her hand as she led the prayer. At the end of the prayer, she verbally "washed us with Christ's blood." We respectfully said, "Amen," and she thanked us. As I left the room, I felt sincerity in my support for her. I did not feel that I had compromised my own spiritual beliefs, but instead, had honored hers. In that moment, I also hoped that someone, regardless of their faith, would one day offer the same compassion and support to my family in their time of need.

As a palliative care pharmacist, I deeply value the contribution of my chaplain colleagues in assessing patients' values and helping to align their treatment accordingly. We cared for a 66-year-old woman with advanced metastatic colorectal cancer and intractable pelvic pain who was admitted to the hospital from home hospice. She had shared with our chaplain her Buddhist spiritual beliefs, which prioritized maintaining mental clarity. These beliefs influenced her and her family's reluctance to use sedating medications, including opioids. After several failed attempts to control the patient's pain, the team, including physicians, a pharmacist, and a chaplain, worked together to consider other options. In the end, the pain anesthesia team initiated a low-dose bupivacaine epidural. This intervention provided significant pain relief while preserving the patient's lucidity, honoring her spiritual priorities.[3] The case highlights how chaplaincy can offer essential insight into patient values, guiding clinical decisions and improving treatment adherence and outcomes at the end of life.

As a palliative care chaplain, I (Kestenbaum) am grateful for the many times that I have visited a seriously ill patient with an interprofessional team, including a pharmacist. Patients often comment on the unlikely pairing but express relief for the opportunity to receive expertise in mind, body, and spiritual approach to palliating their pain and other symptoms. One scenario where the pharmacist–chaplain duo has proven particularly effective is with seriously ill patients with a history of substance use disorder who are now sober but experiencing very real pain from their disease and side effects from treatment that are devastating their quality of life. There are medications that can help, but they are fearful and reluctant to use them because of their history with substance use disorder. On many occasions, I have seen patients underutilize pharmacological approaches or adjust their medications without proper guidance from the medical team, because they fear slipping back into overusing the substance.

Many see addiction, in part, as a spiritual illness.[4] This is why many people are drawn to recovery programs that include "12-Step Spirituality." As a chaplain, I can easily diagnose spiritual suffering that is related to addiction, and I can encourage patients to acknowledge their higher power and empower them to be accountable for their choices. I can remind them that humility has deep spiritual meaning and encourage them to voice their concerns with trust, so the pharmacists can listen with understanding and help shape a treatment plan that eases their fears.

Clinical pharmacists, even when working independently, can play a meaningful role in supporting patients' spiritual needs as "generalists" by recognizing and respecting values that influence treatment decisions. At the same time, pharmacists can serve as advocates for involving chaplaincy "specialists," especially when a patient's beliefs or goals of care suggest the need for deeper spiritual assessment. Even when a pharmacist is the first to encounter these concerns, recognizing the value of specialist spiritual care can lead to more holistic, patient-centered outcomes.

References

1. Gallagher A. Education curricula need to incorporate whole-person care beyond electives. *Pharmacy Times*. Published July 21, 2024. https://www.pharmacytimes.com/view/education-curricula-need-to-incorporate-whole-person-care-beyond-electives. Accessed April 20, 2026.
2. Kestenbaum A, Fitchett G, Galchutt P, et al. Top ten tips palliative care clinicians should know about spirituality in serious illness. *J Palliat Med*. 2022;25(2):312-318. https://doi.org/10.1089/jpm.2021.0522
3. Winters KD, Byrne J, Eckholm N, et al. Palliation of intractable cancer-related pain with low-dose epidural bupivacaine. *J Palliat Med*. 2024;27(3):434-437. https://doi.org/10.1089/jpm.2023.0156.
4. Galanter M, Hansen H, Potenza MN. Article commentary: the role of spirituality in addiction medicine: a position statement from the Spirituality Interest Group of the International Society of Addiction Medicine. *Substance Abuse*. 2021;42(3):269-271. https://doi.org/10.1080/08897077.2021.1941514

Vulnerability in Suffering

Angela Baalmann
PharmD, MS, BCACP

My last advanced pharmacy practice experience (APPE) rotation in transitions of care was the most impactful of all. I was assigned to a large, academic medical center designated as a tertiary and quaternary teaching hospital with nearly 1,000 beds. My daily tasks were to perform medication intake and reconciliations for newly admitted patients and discharge counseling for patients across several inpatient units. Although I felt confident in the educational progress I had made during my fourth year of pharmacy school, the variety of challenges that this rotation presented made me a bit timid with most of my patients.

One day, I was assigned to provide discharge counseling for an adult, female patient with a long-standing history of heart failure who was being discharged from the cardiac hospital wing. Her hospital stay for heart failure exacerbation was relatively short, and only minor medication changes had been made. I entered the patient's room and began to review with her the many educational points inherent in heart failure pharmacologic and nonpharmacologic management. She was alone, and as time passed during our counseling session, I noticed her apathy toward my words and her treatment plan.

Not long into our conversation, I paused to ask her if she planned to carry out any of the treatment plans once she left the hospital. I studied her and noticed that she seemed angry, tense, and a bit sad. Her responses to my questions conveyed her hopeless feelings toward overcoming her battle with heart failure and hurdles to living a healthy lifestyle. She then began to describe the pain she felt each day, which stemmed from her work, marriage, and family relationships. After a few minutes, she stopped talking and stared blankly at the room. I found myself feeling timid once again. I had encountered apathetic patients before in my fourth-year rotations, but a recent personal experience had led me to change how I approach apathy and hopelessness in every area of my own life, and I felt the urge to share this new understanding with my patient.

My faith background has always been Christianity. Raised as a Roman Catholic, I was taught to rely on faith for all of life's answers and use resources from the Church to do so. I have never let go of my Catholic faith, although I came close during my second year of pharmacy school. Part of the challenge was the difficulty I encountered in engaging patients in discussions of faith and articulating spiritual convictions that were then and are still deeply meaningful to me. Several moments, small and large, increased my faith and drove me to study it with greater intensity during pharmacy school. At the time of this rotation, I was in my fourth year, in the

DOI: 10.37573/9781585287727.005

middle of completing a Catholic bioethics certificate program but had yet to apply its teachings to my role as a student pharmacist. My encounter with this patient seemed like my first chance, but I was still quite timid when faced with my patient's apathy and hopelessness. Should I respond by reiterating the medical facts and recommendations, or should I respond by introducing faith into the conversation?

I decided on the latter and asked the patient if I could discuss my faith in God with her. She agreed, and I pointed to a bracelet I was wearing and had worn since starting my pharmacy program. It had a simple cross. I then proceeded to inform her of my Christian roots and discussed a recent piece of work I had read, one that I felt related to her life and its current challenges.

This work was a letter, written by Saint Pope John Paul II, titled "*Salvifici doloris*." This Latin title translates to "redemptive suffering." In this letter, the Pope discusses in-depth the metaphysical reality of human suffering and presents an interpretation of its meaning. He does so from both a secular, nonreligious perspective, as well as a Catholic Christian perspective. I explained to my patient how the Pope's letter had helped me to understand the purpose and value of suffering like never before. For those who aligned with this interpretation, suffering could be one means by which humans could demonstrate their fortitude and manifest a noble reality.

For instance, as a person reflects on their life, they often are most proud of the times when they kept going, staying strong through the most challenging moments. When life is easy, one is not often called upon to demonstrate their character. However, a challenging life allows one to truly live out their distinctive attributes and show others their unique value in the world. From a Catholic Christian perspective, suffering takes on a redemptive meaning by virtue of its connection to Christ's suffering on the cross. The value of suffering can be compounded for those who believe in this Catholic teaching as they experience an aspect of both human and divine life when engaging with suffering.

After I shared these Catholic teachings in an excited and abbreviated manner, I studied my patient and now noticed engagement and a real emotional response to what I had shared. She began to cry and stated that she had never considered suffering in this way. The suffering she had been through had always seemed meaningless to her. Now, she felt it to be more manageable and purposeful than ever before. She professed her belief that God had sent me into her life to send her this message to help save her from this low point in her life. We talked for almost an hour about her life, relationships, and personal journey of faith as a Christian.

Eventually, I asked if I could depart to attend to other patients, and if I could pray with her prior to leaving. She agreed, and I led us through a vocal prayer, asking for God to impart grace into her life, guide her through her continued periods of suffering, and afford her the strength to endure it. I never saw her again but included her in my daily personal prayers throughout the rotation and continue to pray for her now as a pharmacist. The bracelet that I had worn that day remained on my wrist throughout the remainder of my fourth year and first year of residency training, and it provided me with comfort during several moments of my own suffering. It somehow brought me more strength given that it helped make my encounter with this patient possible.

I have told this story to many family members and friends. It is a deeply personal story of mine given what transpired, how it made me feel, and the comfort that it brought to me years after. The manner in which my patient's disposition and our relationship changed still astounds me. I am also amazed at how one symbol, one letter, and one encounter can make all the difference. I remain deeply grateful that my patient allowed me to share my faith and to experience hers during such a vulnerable moment. I now strive to never take such vulnerability for granted in my patients.

I continue to study the intersection of faith and medicine and my role as a pharmacist. Now I often look for the patient's religious background when reviewing their medical records, and I have learned of the presence of chaplains and clinical ethicists in hospitals. I have completed a Master of Science in bioethics since this event and seek to impart what I have learned in my current role as an assistant professor at a school of pharmacy. I hope to influence future pharmacists in a positive manner by reminding them of the vital role that faith plays in many medical encounters, decisions, and relationships. I want future pharmacists to honor the vulnerability inherent in this area of their patients' lives and be brave in being vulnerable themselves should their patient ask for or require it. As Christ said, "*Whatever you did for one of these least brothers of mine, you did for me*" (Matthew 25:40, New American Bible [NAB]).

What About Forgiveness? A Reflection on the Spiritual Practice of Listening

Jake Blair
PharmD, CTHC

In 2018, I was working as a pharmacist in an ambulatory care diabetes clinic. We operated out of a small consultation room in a rural medical facility. We offered diabetes screenings, education, medication therapy management, and connected patients with specialists and other resources. Many of the patients who came to me for screening were at the clinic for some other reason and were either referred to me by their primary care physician or saw our sign in the waiting room and stopped by for a free blood glucose test while they waited.

One morning, a woman in her late 50s came in for a diabetes screening. Her fasting glucose was within normal range. It was ten points higher than it had been just 9 months earlier at a previous screening, and this troubled her. I reassured her that minor fluctuations like this were perfectly normal and were nothing to worry about, but she remained uneasy.

"But what else do I need to do to make sure I don't get diabetes?" she asked, her brow furrowed.

We talked about nutrition, exercise, and weight management. Her body mass index (BMI) was normal, and her overall profile didn't raise any concerns. But the tension in her voice and the anxious questions suggested to me that something else was going on.

She mentioned having chronic gastroesophageal reflux and stomach pain that had persisted for years despite medications and dietary changes. That gave me an idea.

"You seem very worried," I said.

"I worry about a lot of things," she replied. Her voice quivered. Her eyes didn't quite meet mine. I asked a few open-ended questions, and slowly, she began to open up. She told me about how her parents had died very young. As she shared more of her story, layers of grief and regret began to surface—resentment because they were taken too soon and guilt that she hadn't treated them the way she wished she had when they were alive.

DOI: 10.37573/9781585287727.006

"It sounds like this is really weighing on you," I said, wondering if anxiety from this family situation was exacerbating her gastrointestinal problems. "Is there someone you can talk to about all of this?"

"I've been to psychologists, but they haven't helped," she said. "And my last conversation with a priest didn't go well."

I paused for a few seconds, unsure of what to say next. In the stillness of the moment, one word came to mind—forgiveness. It wasn't something I reasoned through. It felt more like an inner prompting, maybe the Holy Spirit.

"What about forgiveness?" I asked, uncertain myself what that really meant.

Her eyes filled with tears. "But how can they forgive me? They passed away years ago." She was talking about her late parents.

Thinking of my own daughter and the unconditional love I have for her, I asked, "If your parents were here today, do you think they would forgive you? Or would they want you to keep being this hard on yourself?"

She was quiet for a second. Then, in a whisper but with certainty: "They would definitely forgive me."

In that moment, I believe she forgave herself. Years of guilt seemed to lift, and the peace in the room was palpable. I asked if she'd like to pray, and she nodded. Prayer deepened our connection as we lifted her burden together. When our visit concluded, she hugged me tightly. It felt like quiet confirmation that I hadn't imagined it all, and that she too felt the peace and connection.

As a pharmacist, I feel equipped to talk about disease states and medications, but I'm not as confident about entering into spiritual conversations with patients. But that day taught me something important: offering spiritual care doesn't require having all the answers ahead of time. It requires attentive listening to the patient. In this case, listening to my patient revealed a wound for which forgiveness was the remedy. I would not say that every ailment is unforgiveness in disguise. Every patient's needs are different. What I can offer is a listening ear and a humble willingness to be a connection between those who are hurting and the God who heals.

It seems to be getting harder and harder to be a good listener. I can feel technology shortening my attention span. What's more, there's increasing pressure in healthcare for greater speed and efficiency in patient encounters. I often feel hurried and distracted by the fast-paced environment, and I struggle to slow down and give my patients the time and attention that they deserve. Listening is a skill worth cultivating, however inefficient, because true healing may depend on being truly heard.

Reflecting on this particular patient encounter reminds me to slow down and be sensitive to the invisible burdens that my patients carry. We must not overlook the emotional and spiritual layers of patient care. Shame, resentment, and loneliness won't show up on any lab results, but they can be significant barriers to health. I continue to rely on and refer patients to those who are professionally trained in counseling and pastoral care, but I believe that pharmacists, too, can be agents of spiritual healing by practicing the simple discipline of listening. I aspire to listen well—to my patients' stories and to the Spirit's still, small voice within me.

An Act of Compassion and Humanity for a Patient at the End of Life

Matthew D. Clark
PharmD

I am a clinical pharmacist at a large academic cancer institution where I have the privilege of working with a multidisciplinary team on an acute palliative care unit where we care for patients at the end of life.

Pharmacy school was filled with in-depth lectures followed by intense, hands-on learning experiences during clinical rotations. I absorbed many aspects of medicine, including pharmacology, pharmacokinetics, and disease state management. Spirituality, however, was not part of the curriculum during my time in pharmacy school. Interestingly, it would be my spirituality, along with my strong Catholic faith, that would lead me to pursue a career in palliative care pharmacy.

When I reflect on my training and personal values, many thoughts come to mind. I grew up in the Roman Catholic faith in the heart of the "Bible Belt," which presented challenges in my predominantly Protestant community. My choice of religious denomination was often disparaged, but it only made my faith stronger.

One influential figure who strengthened me in my faith was my grandfather. He taught me many Catholic prayers, how to pray the Holy Rosary, and was even my sponsor for my confirmation in the Church.

During pharmacy school, my grandfather was diagnosed with adenocarcinoma of the lung, a cancer to which he would eventually succumb. The news hit me harder than a freight train as I never imagined someone so close to me would ever be diagnosed with cancer. Until it happened. Even with a grim prognosis and difficult cancer journey, he remained steadfast in the Lord as well as the Church. I carried this admiration with me through school, residency, and into my role as a palliative care clinical pharmacist.

Providing evidence-based recommendations, calculating safe opioid doses, and serving as a drug information expert are just a few of my daily responsibilities. Everything I am trained to do was, in a sense, routine. That is, until I encountered a young woman during rounds who was experiencing extreme spiritual distress at the end of her life.

DOI: 10.37573/9781585287727.007

This young woman in her early 20s was diagnosed with metastatic adenocarcinoma of the stomach with metastases to the liver, lungs, and bone. She was admitted through the emergency department at our cancer center with sepsis secondary to cholangitis. Through imaging, it was determined that her metastatic disease had progressed significantly, and no further oncologic treatment was warranted. After discussion with the patient and her mother, we decided to transfer her to the palliative care unit (PCU) for comfort measures.

Upon her arrival to the PCU, the mother expressed concern over her daughter's level of comfort. Particularly, she told us that she was afraid that her daughter's symptoms would not be adequately managed at home once she transitioned to hospice. The patient's most burdensome symptoms were pain and dyspnea, and we started her on a morphine patient-controlled analgesia (PCA) pump. We made several dose titrations of the PCA until her pain and dyspnea were relieved. The patient and her mother expressed a reliance on their faith in God, and we requested a visit from the on-site Catholic priest.

While the priest was visiting with the patient and her mother, we were beginning our daily multidisciplinary rounds. With my clinically focused mind, I performed my duties as a pharmacist and monitored her daily opioid usage and made recommendations for dose adjustments. I used all of my training as a pharmacist to keep her comfortable at the end of life, concentrating on what I could accomplish through medicine. However, what I failed to realize was that there was a deeper, nonpalpable reason for her distress. The pain that this patient was experiencing was spiritual in nature.

This became clear when the priest approached our team during rounds. He explained that although this young patient had been raised in the Catholic Church, she had yet to receive the sacraments of baptism and confirmation. He was searching for a team member who was a confirmed Catholic to assist with celebrating these sacraments for the patient prior to her passing. I, being a confirmed Catholic, volunteered.

I entered the room with the priest, unsure what to expect. By this time, our young patient was minimally responsive except for noticeable grimacing and groaning. Her mother was at the bedside in tears seeing her daughter lying in distress. On the table beside the bed lay a rosary and a photo of the patient's brother. With the patient's minimally responsive state, it was difficult for her to recognize these objects that had once brought her peace. This exacerbated her mother's distress. The priest then baptized the daughter with me as her godfather. Subsequently, he confirmed the patient into the Catholic faith with me as her confirmation sponsor.

After receiving these sacraments, the patient rested peacefully. I stayed behind with the patient and her mother after the priest left the room. The mother was still tearful. However, these tears were no longer a result of fear. Instead, they were tears of gratitude. She repeatedly thanked me for my involvement in helping her daughter receive the sacraments. Our conversation quickly shifted from all things medical. We spoke of dreams and ambitions the patient had prior to her illness. She loved to play basketball, and before she was diagnosed with cancer, she was on track to receive a scholarship to play in college. We spoke of the importance of family, and the mother expressed the patient's wish to be surrounded by family members when she passes. These nonclinical conversations seemed to bring peace to her mother's mind after our spiritual encounter. Throughout our conversation, I noticed that the patient no longer was grimacing or moaning in distress.

Her pain and dyspnea soon subsided, and no additional dose adjustments to her PCA were required. Her mother, once again, expressed gratitude for the sacraments the patient received during her stay in the PCU. The patient was then rotated to a nonparenteral regimen of opioids and transitioned home with hospice where she passed away peacefully surrounded by family.

This experience highlights the importance of treating the patient as a whole in palliative care. As healthcare providers, we tend to focus on objective measures without considering the nonmedical factors that can lead to a patient's distress. Aside from viewing the patient's religious affiliation in the demographics section, there aren't many areas in the electronic medical records that assess a patient's spiritual needs. Fortunately, our multidisciplinary team includes a palliative care chaplain who documents their encounters with each patient daily. Without this, it would be difficult to assess the extent that a patient's spiritual distress contributes to their overall symptom burden.

The values of my Catholic faith instilled in me by my grandfather came to fruition during this spiritual encounter. The prayers and rituals that I once took for granted found their way into patient care, bringing peace to a young woman at the end of her life as well as to her mother. This brought them more comfort than any medication could in this situation. In that moment, I replaced my pharmacist cap with one I never thought I would wear during my professional career—a spiritual one. Most importantly, I learned that at the end of life, spiritual care can supersede clinical care, even when the spiritual care is provided by a pharmacist.

Throughout my career, I had tried my best to separate my work life from my personal life. In other words, I would attempt to leave work at work and home at home. Contrarily, this encounter challenged that boundary that I had set for myself. Since this encounter, I have found myself praying the Rosary in the hospital chapel just as I would at home. I look for guidance from God through praying the Rosary when I am faced with difficult patient encounters. As a result, just like the patient and mother in this encounter who felt at peace after receiving the sacraments, I too feel at peace and can carry out my duties as a pharmacist.

Love, Hope, Pharmacy, and Sisters

Melissa M. Corrigan
BS Pharm, CAE, FAPhA, FASHP

Pharmacy is a profession that combines science, clinical skills, and human connections. Many people also believe there is something else in healthcare that addresses the spirit. Early leadership training in an empowering all-girls Catholic high school formed the foundation for my approach to whole-person care. As a teenager, I learned that God is in the details.

The stage was set for me to pursue pharmacy as a career during my high school experience at a Catholic all-girls high school in Illinois. Founded by a Catholic Franciscan sister, the high school eventually combined with a boys' school. After focusing on education, the Franciscan sisters moved north where the community recognized the great need for a hospital when a devastating tornado hit the town. The Franciscan sister then joined forces with a physician and his two sons to plan and staff a hospital that was financially supported by the Franciscan sisters.

My high school experience at the Academy focused on academic excellence and celebrated leadership for young women. This environment gave me the confidence to lead and serve through life first as a student pharmacist and then as a pharmacy practitioner at a nationwide chain of community pharmacies where I worked at 52 pharmacies in just 1 year! After my experience in chain community pharmacy, my interest in serving the pharmacy profession broadened and I completed the American Pharmacists Association (APhA)/National Council of State Pharmacy Association Executives (NCSPAE) Executive Residency in Association Management in Washington, DC. That crucial APhA residency prepared me for a career as a pharmacy association executive. My next step was then founding and leading the Pharmacy Technician Certification Board (PTCB) as an empowered 28-year-old pharmacy leader. During its first three decades, PTCB certified more than 840,000 pharmacy technicians. My career after PTCB evolved to focus on workforce issues, innovation and equity initiatives, and eventually to lead the formation of the American Association of Colleges of Pharmacy's Transformation Center. My foundational education from the sisters of the Academy helped me over time to navigate collaborative environments and provide empathetic care throughout my career journey.

The themes of service in pharmacy and of providing whole-person care were also supported by another sister who became one of my healthcare heroes, Sister M. Gonzalez Duffy. She served as President of the American Society of Hospital Pharmacists, now the American Society of Health-System Pharmacists (ASHP), from 1978 to1979 as the first woman and only religious leader elected to that office.

DOI: 10.37573/9781585287727.008

Sister Gonzalez served as president of ASHP's Research and Education Foundation from 1979 to 1980. She was a member of the ASHP Board of Directors from 1966 to 1969 and 1977 to 1980. In her 1971 Harvey A.K. Whitney Lecture, celebrating ASHP's highest honor, Sister Gonzalez shared, "The emotional side of the sick must never be overlooked." As a pharmacist leader she later added, "So it is *just* because of our increased contact with patients, physicians, and nurses—but mostly patients—that we need to rethink the importance of our personal contributions. We are no longer handling bottles and things but *people*. And people, not things, engender problems; people need help, appreciate care, and recognize *love*. Yes, *love* at its purest and most unselfish, most precious best." (The emphasis on the key words *just*, *people*, and *love* is mine.) In looking back as far as 1971, we see that spirituality in pharmacy is not new. More than 50 years ago, Sister Gonzalez encouraged pharmacists to promote meaning, peace, hope, and love. Her message of presence and providing emotional support, along with the medications, still resonates within me and is ever so relevant today.

Connection is also critically important in healthcare. For patients, connecting with someone in healthcare usually involves some faith, or even hope. Connection supports trust and better patient outcomes. Relationships matter and help us to navigate powerful emotions during illness, tragedy, and grief.

When I was Executive Director/CEO of PTCB, we advocated for national certification, regulation, and education and training for pharmacy technicians. Early in my leadership tenure, I gained tremendous insights on accredited pharmacy technician training programs from Sister Mary Louise Degenhart. A longtime ASHP team member in the Accreditation Services Division, she was the 2016 Whitney medalist and contributed to the Whitney legacy with her published paper, "Pharmacy: Profession of Hope." I found Sister Mary Louise to be a true inspiration, and PTCB was always committed to a strong pharmacy workforce, patient care, and safety.

My leadership at PTCB was heavily influenced by Sister Mary Louise in my support of legislation following a tragic event that captured the interest of the pharmacy profession and society. I will never forget Emily Jerry, a beautiful 2-year-old who died of a preventable medication error that involved a pharmacy technician and a pharmacist. At the time of Emily's death, Ohio was not registering pharmacy technicians, and there were no training or licensing requirements for the role. Chris and Kelly Jerry established the Emily Jerry Foundation and advocated for Emily's law. The law established minimum standards for pharmacy technicians, including age, registration with the State Board of Pharmacy, and passing a competency exam. It also addressed pharmacy technician training, education, criminal records, and disciplinary actions. I reflected on my high school education, Sister Mary Louise's passion, and other professional training that influenced the importance of building authentic, respectful relationships. Emily's story and connecting with Chris Jerry helped me to share the human side of healthcare in my advocacy. PTCB's standards and our support of policies to prevent errors served as an unwavering commitment to save lives.

Bridging science and the soul is an ongoing journey. I reflect on my days at the Academy and my curiosity in biology and organic chemistry that contributed to my career choice of pharmacy. I had a full-circle experience in the past few years when I traveled to a major academic medical center not as a pharmacy leader, but as a caregiver for a family member. My time there produced a range of emotions—joy for being at an internationally known hospital in the world and fear for what was coming next. Then, I found some hope and strength in the lobby when I saw a familiar face, a portrait of the sister who had originally established the Academy! As I contemplated her portrait, I smiled, gathered courage, and thought about the values that have been with me throughout my life and pharmacy career. This religious connection helped me to navigate the healthcare system for my loved one with compassion, resilience, and hope.

Sisters, and their faith and love exhibited in healthcare and pharmacy, have contributed significantly both to my career and to our profession. Many Catholic sisters have made meaningful contributions as trained pharmacists while working with patients and within healthcare institutions. I feel blessed to follow the inspiring examples set by these dedicated women of faith.

Although I no longer provide direct patient care, my faith has informed my career as a management executive and servant-leader. Organizational policies and processes are developed and implemented that support providers who provide spiritual care to our patients and build community with other healthcare practitioners. My education and training, especially my high school experience at a Catholic school, provided the foundation for me to pursue a career in pharmacy. It is important to me that pharmacy providers are encouraged to address mind, body, and spirit in our patients and to pursue collaboration and connection with other healthcare providers. As a mentor, I would advise student pharmacists or emerging leaders interested in incorporating more spiritual care into their practice and training to practice with compassion and empathy.

A Prescription for Hope

Kate Cozart
MEd, PharmD, BCPS, BCGP, BCACP

I practice in a community-based outpatient clinic and conduct dozens of visits per week to focus on chronic disease states and preventative care. I often receive referrals for comprehensive medication management for patients with diabetes, hypertension, hyperlipidemia, tobacco cessation, and weight loss. In my practice, I tend to utilize a "4M" approach to patient care by focusing first on what matters to the patient, and then the other 3 Ms (mentation, mobility, and medications). I also intentionally practice behaviors that are associated with compassion, such as sitting side-by-side with patients, providing nonverbal communication of caring, and offering verbal statements of validation.

In March 2019, I received a new referral for diabetes management. I had no idea how much this 72-year-old gentleman and I would influence one another.

During our first visit, it was obvious that what mattered at that moment was simply for him to be seen. He wasn't a number, and he wasn't just a veteran or a patient with diabetes. He was a grieving widower. He tearfully shared about his wife who had lost her battle with cancer. I provided supportive listening and let him know that he was safe to talk about whatever he needed to with me. He expressed faith that she is in a better place, and I did a quick chart review of the demographics of his patient profile, which confirmed that he identified as a Christian. He proceeded to talk openly that day about his hope in Jesus and his hope to see loved ones again. I also shared with him that I identify as a Christian and that my favorite verse from the Bible at the time was "*The Lord is close to the brokenhearted; he rescues those whose spirits are crushed*" (Psalm 34:18, New Living Translation Version [NLT]).

This conversation of grief with hope and faith continued regularly over the months and years that followed, as he became accustomed to the normalcy of discussing difficult things. We also have openly discussed our shared grief and hope on the anniversaries of his wife's passing and my miscarriage. We both have found comfort in being able to speak freely about these parts of our lives, despite the initial intention that our conversations would focus only on the clinical aspects of his care.

I have no doubt that his trust in me as a clinician was impacted positively that day and for the several years we have worked together since, because he was able to see that I work as a pharmacist to honor God and not just to please an employer. He was also able to see that my recommendations regarding treatment were through the lens of seeing him as a person, a loved child of God, and not just a number. He

DOI: 10.37573/9781585287727.009

continues to know to this day that if I make a clinical recommendation, it is because I truly believe it is the best option for him and that I will never approach decisions with any other mindset than shared decision-making. Over the years, we have also made significant progress toward the health goals that matter to him, including minimizing his hypoglycemia risk and choosing medications that are most appropriate for all of his chronic disease states.

He found that he can trust me with hard conversations from the very first day. After some time, he was able to admit to me that his binge-eating behavior occasionally stems from guilt over removing his wife from life support. Over the years, we have had extensive talks about her prognosis and his decision, in addition to her life and their marriage, and I have always been a compassionate ear, offering nonverbal communication of caring as he processes those feelings. As he talks more freely about his emotions and experiences, a level of accountability has been added to our relationship that can only be built from a place of vulnerability.

My time caring for this now 78-year-old gentleman has impacted me personally in a very profound way. As I continued to care for him, I started to see my own identity as a spiritual person as an integral part of my professional disposition as a pharmacist. I am very active as a writer and speaker on healthy well-being where I address topics, such as burnout and professional identity. I believe in the idea that a strong sense of professional identity helps mitigate burnout, and that one of the three facets of burnout is a reduced sense of personal accomplishment. I present an alternative argument that personal accomplishment is not our goal any longer. What if every accomplishment and achievement as a clinician or professional is not viewed as "mine" at all, but a reflection of God as my creator? When I find confidence in Him as the one responsible for "my" victories or accomplishments, my light isn't tempted to burn out from lack of personal accomplishment. Instead, I choose to root my identity and light in whose I am.

This also impacted me as a professional in that it encouraged me to recognize and respond not only to opportunities for compassion, but also for spiritual comfort. It is not something that I observed often from my own mentors, so the concept was novel to me. However, sometimes patients are looking for just that—a provider who cares about their spiritual health in addition to the physical. When conversations are initiated by patients, I no longer shy away from discussions of faith and have had the opportunity to let students see what it looks like for a provider to provide excellent patient care within the context of spirituality and faith. It isn't every day that I have discussions about grief and hope with my patients, but I for one am grateful for the days when I do get to be part of those conversations and we see the light in one another's shared humanity.

The interaction described above made a world of difference in the trust between this patient and me as his provider. He was able to have conversations with me much more easily, because he knew that I would not judge him and would be comfortable providing spiritual support. I believe that providing spiritual care is a necessary part of whole-person care and that if done within the context of the patient's comfort, it is an excellent role for any clinician or pharmacist. I believe that letting patients talk openly about faith with me, or feel comfortable asking me for prayer, allows us to know we have common ground and love for each other as brothers and sisters. This essay also highlights that my place as a Christian is a vital part of the professional work that I do in caring for others.

The Fate of Faith: Lessons from a Hospital Encounter

Jeremy Espeut
PharmD, MBA, MS

One particular interaction forever shaped how I approach patients, not only as bodies in need of healing but as whole persons with spiritual lives that sometimes speak louder than their physical symptoms. It occurred during my advanced pharmacy practice experiences (APPEs) in my final year of pharmacy school on one of my inpatient hospital rotations. Although my faith has been central to my life from my earliest days, I often found it was one of the unspoken "taboo" subjects in school and on clinical rotations, much like politics. In lecture halls and professional discussions, conversations about religion and spirituality were avoided, as if acknowledging personal belief might somehow compromise objectivity or professionalism. Although many of my peers held deep convictions, faith was seldom mentioned, and spirituality rarely surfaced in our coursework or clinical discussions. I learned quickly that within academic settings, it was safer to leave matters of faith at the door.

During my APPE experience, I was assigned to talk with a patient before they went home about adherence to the DASH (Dietary Approaches to Stop Hypertension) diet and other lifestyle modifications to treat his high blood pressure. I walked into his room prepared with the usual counseling points, such as reduced sodium intake, moderation of red meat, and an emphasis on eating fruits, vegetables, and whole grains. I didn't think at all about engaging him in a conversation about his spirituality.

Halfway through my carefully rehearsed counseling session, the patient interrupted me. He listened politely, then leaned forward with a quiet intensity.

"Listen," he said, "I worked hard throughout my life to live a certain lifestyle. And I believe in *Qadar*. Do you know what *Qadar* is?" I paused. The word was unfamiliar, although I noticed the Qur'an on his bedside table, a detail that I had registered but not yet integrated into the conversation. I admitted that I did not know, and he graciously explained.

"*Qadar*," he said, "is divine destiny. It is Allah's decree, the belief that all things unfold according to God's will. My health, my challenges, my very life are guided by *Qadar*. You talk to me about completely changing my diet and doing exercise, but I know that ultimately, God has already written my story."

DOI: 10.37573/9781585287727.010

It would have been easy to retreat, to say nothing further of faith, and continue listing more low-sodium food substitutions. But instead, I leaned into the conversation. I acknowledged his belief in *Qadar* and gently connected it with my own understanding of God's providence as a Christian. I did not try to persuade him to adopt my theology; rather, I expressed respect for his conviction and a recognition that our beliefs, although expressed differently, both spoke to a trust in divine order. South Florida is a melting pot, home to people from every cultural and religious background. It is not unusual to see a patient's rosary beads draped over a bed rail, a Torah tucked into a bag, or a Qur'an open on a nightstand. Yet too often, providers overlook these signs. We are trained to examine medication lists and lab values, but not necessarily the spiritual cues that reveal a patient's deeper worldview and give us a window to incorporate it into our standard of care.

That day, the Qur'an at the bedside was not just a book; it was an invitation. My encounter with this patient made me far more attentive to these cues. Now in practice within a faith-based health system, I carry that awareness with me daily. Spiritual care is not an add-on; it is part of whole-person care. The conversation with my patient also raised profound questions about the intersection of fate and responsibility. As healthcare providers, we promote lifestyle modifications, adherence, and evidence-based practices. We must recognize that many patients hold spiritual convictions that interpret illness and healing through the lens of divine will.

Some might see fatalism in his words: "God has written my story, so why change my diet?" But I did not hear resignation. I heard trust. He was not indifferent to my counsel; rather, he was framing it within his theology of destiny. His conviction challenged me to present lifestyle recommendations, not as a denial of divine will, but as a way of honoring the life and health that God had entrusted to him. My patient taught me to soften my approach to patient interactions, and I became more comfortable asking gentle, open-ended questions that invite patients to share what mattered most to them spiritually. Sometimes the clues are visible, such as a Qur'an or rosary; other times, they emerge only after trust has been established, or sometimes not at all, which is also completely okay. I've learned to listen for more than physical symptoms. I listen for faith.

The encounter reminded me that respect opens doors. My willingness to admit ignorance about Islam and *Qadar* created space for the patient to teach me, and in turn, that respect fostered dialogue and built trust. I also discovered that faith itself can serve as a common language. Even across different religions, themes of divine guidance, destiny, and trust create bridges that strengthen the provider–patient relationship. I came to understand that whole-person care requires spiritual awareness. Pharmacists cannot treat only the body; to ignore spirituality is to overlook a dimension of the patient's reality that often shapes adherence, motivation, and healing. In emphasizing social determinants of faith, healthcare teams recognize that a patient's health outcomes are not defined solely by their lab values or prescriptions but also by factors, such as access to nutritious food, stable housing, reliable transportation, and emotional support systems. I recognized that faith systems directly influence health decisions. When I appreciate a patient's belief system, I can contextualize my advice so that it resonates as not only clinically sound but also personally meaningful.

I entered pharmacy because I wanted to promote healing. What I continue to learn is that healing is not only physical; it is spiritual. My upbringing in faith and my faith today are not separate from my role as a pharmacist. They are interwoven.

Spiritual activities keep me grounded, reminding me that my work is a vocation, not just a job. Integrating spiritual awareness allows me to provide care that is compassionate, respectful, and truly whole-person centered.

A Redirected Calling

Diane B. Ginsburg
PhD, MS, RPh, FASHP, DASPL

I practiced in Texas in health-system pharmacy and currently practice in academia with an expertise in pharmacy law and bioethics. However, completing a pharmacy residency and a master's degree after earning my pharmacy degree were highly influential for me, largely due to the strong mentorship of my program director. He was deeply committed to providing leadership not only to the residents but also to the broader professional pharmacy community. I attribute my strong affinity for encouraging and engaging with young pharmacy students and new practitioners, in part, to his mentorship.

In guiding students to reflect on their professional values and responsibilities to both patients and colleagues, I often consider how my Jewish background has influenced my perspective. I think about the evolution of what I believe and value, and how my personal growth in beliefs and values continues to influence the pharmacy students I recruit and mentor.

I grew up in an orthodox home until my grandfather passed away when I was 10 years old. My grandmother, who was born in Kiev and immigrated to the United States when she was in her teens, took a stronger role in shaping our religious life. She was what I would consider to be a "ritualist." The rituals of Judaism were important to her, and she held tightly to the traditions she had grown up with in Ukraine; frequently, her opinions and actions within Judaism followed her orthodox upbringing. But she never really shared what the faith meant to her personally. One example that impacted me was not being permitted to study and become a bat mitzvah like Jewish boys did. Even Sunday school wasn't about learning the tenets of my religion but to learn the rituals that I would be expected to follow.

My grandmother was not active in our synagogue, and the importance of giving back to one's community was not instilled in me by her or my parents. We were somewhat observant during the high holidays (Rosh Hashanah and Yom Kippur), but it was the rituals themselves—what we do during those holidays, not their profound meanings—that were emphasized.

My parents stressed that education was the most important thing in one's life. I was expected to be a high achiever and to never settle for anything less than the highest grades. Failure was never a word used in my home. I do not recall how the emphasis on achievement was in any way attributed to the spiritual aspects of my religion. I did as I was expected and taught by my parents and grandparents—graduate from high school and start college a year early, be a high-achieving student,

DOI: 10.37573/9781585287727.011

pursue graduate education, and be a success within my profession. None of these things are negative, and I greatly appreciated these values being instilled in me.

I have spent my career giving back to the profession that I love, never shying away from opportunities where I could contribute. Many times, programs and meetings would be scheduled during the Jewish High Holidays, and I have attended and participated in meetings and conferences at the expense of my religion. As someone of the Jewish faith, I have always been in the minority in professional settings. However, I knew that if I wanted to continue to succeed in my career, I would need to attend and participate. When I would ask and/or mention that a conference or meetings were being held during the holidays, I would frequently hear, "Oh, we didn't realize this. We will do a better job with planning next year." Even today, this still occurs on a frequent basis.

In my role as an educator, I often had students ask for permission to miss class or reschedule exams because of religious holidays. My grandmother had instilled in me the importance of respecting people, no matter their faith, so I always grant their requests. I worked with the students to ensure that they could fully practice their faith without penalty. For me, it was also an opportunity—I would take the time to learn about the holiday, its place in their tradition, and what it meant to them personally. What stood out most was how deeply their faith shaped their core values, something clearly demonstrated in their actions.

As someone who teaches biomedical ethics, the role of religion in health care is prominent. Patients and their families make decisions influenced by their faith. As my students and I review patient cases, we discuss what role religion plays in our provision of patient care. My students are encouraged to take a holistic view of the patient's situation and examine and apply ethical principles to addressing dilemmas. They are encouraged to view the situation through a lens that considers the faith of both the student themselves and the patient. A key lens to see a situation through is the student's and patient's faith. My hope is that students know this is not something to be dismissed but applied as appropriate to an ethical dilemma.

My husband's family is not very religious; however, they are very philanthropic and are actively involved with the Jewish community in south Texas. I observed them serving in leadership positions within multiple Jewish organizations at all levels. They never questioned me regarding my volunteerism within my profession but would ask what my engagement was within my community, the Jewish community.

My calling has always been to my profession, but I realized as someone in a minority, it was important to give back to my community. If I could give tens of thousands of hours to the pharmacy profession, I could certainly volunteer my time to the Jewish community. I feel that it is critical that I "walk my talk" within my faith as well as my profession. I have served on the board of my synagogue to direct efforts to support our local Jewish community. Through this involvement, I studied and became a bat mitzvah at 31 (and it is much harder to do this when you are an adult in less than a year than how Jewish children prepare).

I have the privilege of serving on the board of directors for Texas Hillel. The mission of Texas Hillel at my university is to "enrich the lives of Jewish undergraduate and graduate students so they can enrich the Jewish people and the world. This is achieved by providing a variety of programs and opportunities, including student leadership development, Jewish life and learning experiences, and support for Israel and global Jewish peoplehood."

In my role on the Hillel Board, I can connect with Jewish students at all levels. I have mentored several undergraduate students who have subsequently applied and been accepted into our PharmD program. I can discuss my "why" behind my decision to become engaged with the Jewish community at my university. My "why" is this redirected calling—the duty and responsibility I feel to contribute and support my community. This has become increasingly important with the rise of antisemitism as threats to the Jewish community in our neighborhoods and our students on campus. My involvement with Texas Hillel has deepened my understanding of the Jewish faith and how we can use the values we learn in our respective religions in the care we provide to our patients and our communities.

Holistic Pharmacist-Led Patient Care in a West African Hospital Setting

Anonymous

Throughout my practice in West Africa, as well as in the United States, I have seen spirituality be the foundation of one's worldview and directly influence how patients manage difficult life circumstances. A patient's spirituality is something that is deeply personal and intimate, often defining who they are, how they present themselves, and influencing their perspective on the world. To provide the best possible patient care, pharmacists need to give attention to an aspect that may be very important to the patient, namely spirituality.

At our hospital, which is known in the region for being a Christian hospital, caring for a patient's spirituality is prioritized, as we see that spirituality is a major component of holistic care. Patients of varying religious backgrounds choose to come to our hospital, expecting to hear the Gospel of Jesus Christ many different times during their hospital visit.

One such patient, an 86-year-old woman, was admitted to the intensive care unit at our small 40-bed mission hospital in rural, French-speaking West Africa. She had breast cancer and congestive heart failure as well as other health issues. Today, she was having trouble breathing, repeatedly coughing, and gasping for breath as her symptoms were not controlled by her medication regimen and oxygen that were started in the emergency department. She sat hunched over, body bent at a 45-degree angle day and night, because it was the only position that would relieve her urge to cough.

As a part of my practice, I provide rounding services with some of the hospital's medical providers. During the initial patient encounter, I asked the worried family if they had been anywhere else for care. Her adult son eagerly said, "Yes, look!" and presented me with notes, x-rays, radiology scans, and an entire grocery bag full of half-taken prescription medications from various healthcare facilities all over the country. Without an electronic medical record or strong lines of communication between facilities, we must get creative as we learn a patient's medical history. After our review of the notes, radiology studies, and medications, it was evident that her cancer and heart failure had progressed beyond the level of care that we, nor any other facility in the country, could provide. Her illnesses were terminal; she was very likely going to die in the upcoming weeks or months. I suspected that instead

DOI: 10.37573/9781585287727.012

of telling the family about the seriousness of her condition, the other facilities may have just discharged her the moment she was well enough to leave.

In this part of Africa, it is culturally appropriate that a family or village representative make all decisions related to the care and end-of-life arrangements for a critically ill relative or neighbor. As a medical team, we decided to talk with the patient's representative, her son, to explain what hospice care was, and how his mother was not going to recover. Our goals were to treat her symptoms and make her comfortable. We also explained that once she began hospice, all her care at the hospital (eg, follow-up visits, medications, laboratory assessments, examinations) would be financially covered by the benevolence fund, because our hospital's hospice program offers comprehensive care at no cost. He appeared gracious, almost relieved, to finally have answers to his mom's health and that someone would walk with them through this process to the end of her life.

After a week as an inpatient, she was discharged with a home hospice plan and a follow-up visit set for 3 weeks later, giving her and her family time to adjust while knowing support was close at hand. Shortly before her scheduled follow-up, the family brought the patient back to the hospital, saying that her breathing had worsened again. Admission to the hospital offered us new opportunities to provide comfort care as well as spiritual care for her and her family.

To provide some context, a chaplain visits each admitted patient daily for a bedside conversation. The hospital chaplains are people from the local community who bring with them the ability to speak several nearby tribal languages and understand all the cultural cues that need to be followed. Should the chaplain or myself encounter someone who doesn't want to speak with us, we honor their request and respectfully offer to speak with them the following day. One morning while rounding with the medical team, I felt inspired to circle back to have a pointed, intentional conversation with this patient. The topic of transitions came to my mind—in her case, the transition from life to death. I found an available chaplain and asked him to come along to translate my French into her family's language.

When I entered the patient's room, I asked the patient's family, her representatives, if I could speak with her about Jesus. They eagerly responded, "Yes, of course!" I started by sharing how all of us have several transitions during our day. For example, I finish getting ready in the morning and "transition" to work. Then, I round on the first patient and "transition" to the second. After work is finished, I "transition" back home where there are other things that I need to do. I used the very familiar idea of transitions to mention that she was very close to a transition herself—the transition from life on this earth to the next world.

After the stage was set and the patient and her family were engaged, I asked the chaplain to share. Knowing that some, but not all, of the family were professing Christians, the chaplain spoke for about 25 minutes about the complete story of creation, the fall when man sinned for the first time, and how God sent his Son, Jesus, as a sacrifice on our behalf to pay the price for all of mankind's sin. He highlighted the teaching found in the Bible, which says "*For it is by grace you have been saved, through faith—and this is not from yourselves, it is the gift of God—not by works, so that no one can boast*" (Ephesians 2:8-9, New International Version [NIV]). Many patients that we encounter believe that they can get to heaven by trying to outweigh bad works with good works. This belief causes many of our patients extreme anxiety when they are near death, wondering if they have done enough good to outweigh the bad. While listening, the patient and her family would stop the chaplain and ask clarifying questions, excitedly waiting for the chaplain's answer. I sat silently. The patient who was previously too weak to look at us or talk was now staring directly at the chaplain with an intense look in her eyes. His talking slowed down, and I sensed that the invitation to follow Jesus was close to the end. Suddenly, there was complete silence throughout the room. All eyes were focused on the patient; too physically weak to talk, hunched over from her illnesses, and yet looking strong and fierce at the same time. With the slight, slow movement of her head, she nodded, "yes."

What followed was the closest thing to a joyful noise I have ever heard. Her one daughter who also professes to be a Christian, suddenly started crying and yelling praises to God. The chaplain with arms raised was praying out loud. The patient sat there, with this strong look in her eyes, seemingly fully cognizant of the decision she had made to follow Jesus.

A week later the patient passed away with her family at her bedside. When I heard the news, I went to them and sat with them, bringing no message or special words to say, but rather copying their actions of mourning and showing my solidarity. This was not a sad death, but rather one of hope. One family member took out his phone and asked if he could take my photo, saying, "I want to tell the village all that you and this hospital have done for us. You have cared for us well." The family gave me their cell phone numbers, saying "Anytime you want to come to our village, you will be an honored guest."

While this interaction deeply impacted the patient on a personal level, this interaction also greatly impacted the family of the patient and their perception of the medical providers at our hospital. The family was visibly distraught over the health of their mom, longing for her health, but they also realized that her time here on earth was limited. As depicted in the narrative, this family responded with such joy, peace, and happiness at their mother's decision to accept the Gospel of Jesus Christ. They did not seem heartbroken when she passed away. Instead, they seemed honored to have been a part of her journey and longed for more people in their village to experience the kindness, care, and compassion displayed by our hospital and providers as we cared for their mom in all aspects of her personhood, including the physical, mental, social, and spiritual.

The Power of Prayer

Elisa Greene

PharmD

Chatter in at least three languages filtered into the consultation room while I met with a patient one morning last spring. We'll call her Maria. We've seen each other almost every month for more than the decade where I've served as an ambulatory care clinical pharmacist at the urban, faith-based community clinic.

I've been privileged to develop long-term relationships with my patients. I love being able to walk alongside them through their lives, to know their joy and sorrow, to connect authentically through shared humanity. Maria's complicated medical history has led to frequent visits, which provide ample opportunity for us to discuss her life, including her Christian faith.

My clinic exists to serve those in need with healthcare that reflects our Christian faith. We bring a whole-person approach to caring for uninsured, underserved, and culturally marginalized individuals. Whole-person care means that the mind, body, soul, and spirit of each person entering our doors are honored and considered during their visits.

Spiritual history-taking is part of our intake process, often using the HOPE model. During new patient visits, we ask everyone where they find sources of *hope* (H), how they engage with *organized religion* (O), what personal *spiritual practices* they use (P), and about the *effects* of their spirituality on their medical care and needs (E). The patient's spirituality guides and supports the care provided by our team.

Although Maria's primary provider took her history, I knew of her Christian faith, because it came up frequently in our previous conversations. The electronic medical record noted "Christian" as part of her social history. Through the conversations across many appointments, I had learned that her husband served as a pastor of a local church. "God willing," she would say, when presented with a plan to relieve her pain. She responded, "Thank you, God," when we found a pharmacy with her backordered prescription in stock.

Over the years, I've walked alongside her as we navigated difficult personal transitions and complicated medical challenges. We've built trust through much trial and error as she patiently tried medications and partnered with me to solve problems until we found something that worked. Hallelujah! We rejoiced that day. We've cried and prayed together in the exam room about fears surrounding her family's circumstances, joy over a new grandchild, frustration with a lack of diagnostic answers, and loneliness in seasons of hardship.

DOI: 10.37573/9781585287727.013

On this particular day, I tried to hide my own heavy emotions, which were restless inside me and on the verge of spilling out. As she was gathering her things to leave, she stopped and sat back down. "*Doctora*," she said gently, "How are *you*? How is your family?"

Moved that she had noticed and taken the time to ask, I shared that my mom had received a difficult diagnosis that week and that I was worried for her. "Oh *Doctora*, I will pray for her," Maria said, switching to her native Spanish and following immediately in prayer, "God, please heal the doctor's mom." Simple. Powerful. Present.

Maria continues to pray for me and my mother. Not a single visit has passed without her asking in an endearing mix of Spanish and English, "*Doctora*, how's your mami?" I continue to be utterly humbled and honored by her generosity in approaching God on my behalf.

A traditional paternalistic healthcare model promotes one-directional healing. The healthcare provider offers resources to help the patient. In a more modern patient-centered care model, the provider supports the patient in identifying and drawing upon their own resources. Focusing on the patient as an actor in their own health instead of merely being a recipient of healing rightly acknowledges that patients can also help themselves. It is a step toward sharing healing power.

Power is a nuanced concept. Power dynamics shape healthcare in complex and subtle ways. Asymmetries pile up at each encounter. I wear the white coat. I hold the knowledge. I control the resources. I wield the authority. Reluctantly, compassionately, generously . . . or not. Anyone who has experienced significant injury or illness knows that being thrust into the position of patient frequently elicits deep discomfort. On the exam table, we experience what it is to be vulnerable, dependent, perhaps even powerless. And powerlessness is only a few steps away from despair.

Earthly power structures *should* exist for good, yet sometimes actually cause harm. In healthcare, we use shared decision-making, cultural humility, trauma-informed care, and other tools to mitigate these harms. We aspire to *empower* the patient, ignoring how that language might implicitly reinforce the power imbalance at play. We aspire to do good. Sometimes, perhaps, we do.

Christians recognize God's power, often praying for it to move on their behalf or on the behalf of loved ones. Maria and I have both found faith in God. Through this spiritual lens, we recognize that although I am the healthcare provider, and she is the patient, God is the one who ultimately heals. Although we both identify as Christians, this belief exists across multiple religious traditions. In the Bible, the book of Exodus 15:26 (New International Version [NIV]) reads, "*I am the Lord, your healer.*" The Jewish *Torah* includes the book of Exodus, and the *Islamic* Quran contains scripture portraying God as the ultimate source of healing (Surah Ash-Shu'ara 26:80).

This worldview that acknowledges God as the ultimate healer upends other perceptions of power and privilege in the best of ways. It reorients us both—provider and patient—to our identities in God, freeing me from needing to have all the answers and enabling Maria to approach the encounter as an equal.

Medically, I have access to innumerable drug information resources, clinical trials, and guideline documents. In every visit, I bring evidence-based recommendations and clinical experience to support her healing. Spiritually, *both* of us have access to the all-powerful, all-knowing divine Healer. *Both* of us can approach Him on behalf of each other. In bringing our resources to serve others, we find that we *both* have full quivers. Sometimes, He uses the healthcare provider and their clinical resources to find the right medicine for the patient. And sometimes, as on this day, He uses the patient and their spiritual resources to find the right words to comfort the heart of the clinician.

My advice to providers who would like to incorporate spiritual care into their practice is that spirituality is a part of every person. Don't be afraid to acknowledge it and dive in; brainstorm questions or statements that would feel authentic to your own spirituality while allowing the patient to be centered in theirs. This doesn't have to be overly religious; it doesn't have to be religious at all. The HOPE model provides a framework that you might find helpful. Simply asking, "What would nourish your spirit right now?" or saying, "I can sense that your spirit feels heavy," could open the door for the patient to share.

Beyond the Guidelines: Practicing the Humanity of Medicine

Kevin Thomas Hatley
PharmD candidate

I am a student pharmacist scheduled to graduate in 2026 after spending 12 years as an emergency medicine technician. I made the change because for me pharmacy is the perfect balance of patient care and subject expertise. I will share how I was able to incorporate spirituality into emergency medicine care as well as how I have been able to incorporate spirituality into the care of patients as a pharmacy student.

The emergency department (ED) sees the entire spectrum of patients, from a patient seeking a medication refill or attention for a hangnail, to one needing cardiopulmonary resuscitation or hospice care. I have had the solemn privilege of being present when patients are at their worst, when they don't know what comes next, or where to turn. In those moments, many patients rely on their spiritual beliefs. Working as an ED technician before pharmacy school, I had many opportunities to address the spiritual aspects of illness and healing.

A patient with memory decline who could no longer live alone stayed in the ED for several days while physicians stabilized her various medical conditions and social workers found placement in a memory care facility. During her stay in the ED, I was often asked to sit with her for the duration of my shift to keep her safe. Her only belongings were her glasses and a Bible. I learned that her Christian faith had always been a significant part of her life, and she was worried about losing that dimension of her life as her condition declined. She was uncomfortable and very anxious in the ED, but the one thing that was comforting to her was reading the Bible. I was able to ease her anxiety not with medication but by reading her favorite parts of the Bible to her. One of the most rewarding moments of my healthcare career was to provide comfort for her as we prayed for healing and peace as she transitioned to a new phase of life.

As a pharmacy student, my interaction with patients has been more limited as I learn pharmacists' responsibilities. My pharmacy school sets up health fairs at senior centers. Recently, I was a counselor for our bone mineral density screening committee. Our process included an extensive interview with the patient and subsequent counseling on factors that might impact bone health or fall risk. The interview included a medical history, a medication history, their diet, and social factors, such as depression, living arrangements, and personal relationships. Inevitably when having conversations about personal matters, patients would also share more

DOI: 10.37573/9781585287727.014

personal factors that provide them with motivation for remaining healthy and preventing fall injuries. Sometimes this included their religious beliefs. A woman whom I was counseling was very vocal about her belief that God was watching out for her and recounted several occasions when she fell or almost fell but was found by chance soon afterward. She told me she feels certain that she will be able to maintain her health, because she does not need to rely only on her own strength, but also the help that comes from God. I was able to have a conversation with her, supporting her in her belief, and encouraging a greater confidence that her health can improve. We discussed that we had developed a health management plan that relied on her participation with God's help.

I feel called to reflect Christ-like compassion toward all patients, regardless of shared beliefs. Being able to make a difference in someone's health by helping them manage their medications is extremely rewarding but so is the ability to positively impact their social and spiritual well-being. We must acknowledge for ourselves and our patients that we are not just physical beings with disease pathologies who can be defined and placed into guidelines. Instead, as a competent practitioner, it is equally important that we support our patients' spiritual well-being along with their physical ailments. I will continue to work toward incorporating this into my practice in my career as a pharmacist. As I continue my journey through pharmacy school and into clinical practice, I remain committed to treating patients as whole persons. My goal is not only to practice evidence-based medicine but also to provide compassionate, faith-sensitive care whenever appropriate. Whether or not patients share my beliefs, I aim to bring empathy, peace, and dignity into every interaction. I would recommend to fellow students and pharmacy colleagues that they take cues from their patients. If the patient speaks of their spirituality, I encourage them to take advantage of the opportunity to connect with the patient on another dimension. As a caregiver, I have found it personally rewarding to establish this deep connection with my patients. My faith is central to my worldview, and engaging with the spiritual side of patient care encourages me to practice pharmacy with empathy and care.

Establishing Patient Credibility in Long-Term Care Through Spirituality

Mark S. Johnson
PharmD, MACE, BCPS

I first met the patient approximately 15 years ago at the local Presbyterian church (USA) where we were both members. We served on several committees together as ruling elders of our church and developed a rapport during that time. She was very active in the church, singing in the choir, serving on numerous church committees, and participating in many other areas of church life. I remember how much enthusiasm, organization, as well as the many ideas and the desire to continually learn that she brought to all that she did, and it was always a pleasure to serve with her. In her mid-70s, she had worked in administrative and managerial positions in the Washington, DC, area prior to her and her husband's retirement.

I became reacquainted with the patient around 3 years ago. As a faculty member at a school of pharmacy, I developed an advanced pharmacy practice experience (APPE) rotation at a local faith-based, nonprofit continuing care retirement community where she and her husband resided. The facility offers a continuum of care for seniors, including independent living, assisted living, memory care, skilled nursing, and acute rehabilitation. The APPE that I developed is called, "Whole Person Care in Pharmacy Practice." Its purpose is to help students gain an appreciation for how a pharmacist can provide whole-person care (treating the patient as a mind, body, and spirit) to older adults and vulnerable populations as a part of an interprofessional team. It is based on the premise that delivering healing and compassionate care for the whole person should be the mission of medicine and healthcare and is supported by an abundance of evidence demonstrating improved patient outcomes when spirituality is incorporated into the care of patients. In addition to providing clinical pharmacy support for the long-term care patients by rounding with the medical and nursing staffs, the APPE students also have weekly meetings with the on-site chaplain and conduct spiritual histories on some of the patients with the chaplain. The primary goals of the APPE are for students to help patients to better understand and explore their disease states and medicines from a clinical and spiritual perspective and appreciate the impact that spirituality might have in their patients' daily lives.

DOI: 10.37573/9781585287727.015

This patient was one of the first patients with whom I interacted as I began my clinical pharmacy practice at the facility. Although I had not seen the patient for several years, our previous work together at church helped us both recognize each other and get reacquainted, particularly as it related to church and spiritual matters. She was now in her early 90s and resided in assisted living. She was still very active but was beginning to have some challenges with her activities of daily living, particularly with managing her medications due to the early stages of dementia. My student pharmacists and I would interact with her when we saw her walking in the facility or coming to the medical clinic for nursing and medical appointments. She took a keen interest in my students and would ask us questions about her medications, including the many supplements and vitamins that she took.

The patient had always managed her medications and supplements but was resistant to giving up control when the medical and nursing staff recommended that they take over responsibility for administering her medications because of her increasing dementia. The medical director, recognizing the spiritual rapport that I had developed with the patient, asked the patient if she would be willing to talk with me and my students about her medications, and she agreed.

The medications were stored in a cabinet in her assisted living room where we discovered multiple herbal supplements, vitamins, and prescription medicines. Many of them were beyond their expiration date or had no solid evidence to support continuation. We went through each individual medicine, supplement, and vitamin with the patient and eliminated the unnecessary ones and expired products. She showed us her meticulous notes and schedules that she recorded on her medications and supplements, but it was evident that she was having difficulty keeping up with it all. The patient was amendable overall to our help and agreed to the plan to have the nursing staff administer her revised and streamlined medicines, supplements, and vitamins. Although she had been reluctant at first, after our review she expressed a sense of relief to not have to bear this responsibility. The medical and nursing staffs were very pleased with this outcome and appreciated the pharmacy intervention.

Several months passed and the patient's dementia progressed, so she was transferred to the memory care unit, where we made rounds with the medical director. Once during rounds, the patient expressed disapproval of our taking some of her supplements away. We gently reminded her of the mutual agreement that we came to when we made the changes. Over time, her disapproval subsided.

She always enjoyed meeting my students, and we continued to visit with her in the memory care unit. Her room was filled with beautiful artwork that she had collected over many years, including pictures of her family and religious pictures and symbols. Her son was a Presbyterian minister, and we listened as she spoke fondly of him, along with her other children and grandchildren as her family was very important to her. All of these items were conversation starters, particularly with one of my students who enjoyed artwork and spent some time with her listening to her describe the various pieces of art and what they meant to her. The student developed such a good rapport with the patient that they received an award in 2024 for Excellence in Caring for Older Adults from the American Society of Consultant Pharmacists.

Several months later, the patient was placed in hospice care due to her deteriorating medical conditions and dementia. Her family was called in to be with her around her bedside. As we rounded on her one day, the medical director asked if I would like to say a prayer over the patient with her family, which I did. I attended her funeral, and the family was very appreciative of the work and support that we all had given to her. The patient's husband was also in the skilled nursing facility at that point, and I visited with him to provide comfort and support. I later continued to visit him on medical and pharmacy rounds and provided both medical and spiritual support to him.

This interaction with the patient has made me realize the value of treating the whole patient. I do not feel that this interaction would have occurred or would have gone as well without first establishing a spiritual connection with the patient. This spiritual connection gave me credibility with her and helped me to earn her trust so that I could take care of her pharmacy needs, even though she sometimes questioned the actions that I recommended. As a result, I felt a much greater sense of fulfillment as a pharmacist.

A Call to Fill the Spiritual Gap in Holistic Care

Kendra A.N. Lucas
PharmD

When spiritual care is not seamlessly integrated into a healthcare system, it can become challenging for both patients and providers to address the subject of spirituality in the context of medical care. As a pharmacist who has practiced in community, specialty, and nonprofit settings, I have firsthand experience regarding the time constraints, company policies, and sensitivities surrounding the topic that often prevent pharmacists from broaching the subject of spirituality. However, in my most recent position as a director of clinical services at a nonprofit healthcare organization, I had the unique opportunity to incorporate spiritual care into daily practice. In doing so, I experienced positive changes in my patients' demeanor and attitude toward their health, a growth in patient trust toward our healthcare team, and an overall sense of belonging by both patients and staff. While I have numerous examples of how spirituality has impacted my life and the lives of my patients, one case in particular stands out to me as the catalyst for transforming how I approach my personal practice.

The organization that I worked at is a 501(c)(3) nonprofit located in Indiana that provides low-cost medical, dental, mental, and spiritual care services to Hoosiers without health insurance. The organization was founded by a Christian church, and all staff and volunteers have declared their Christian faith. However, while the organization is rooted in Christianity, the organization welcomes all uninsured Hoosiers as patients—regardless of religious background. As part of routine care, staff and volunteers offer optional prayer at each appointment, and every clinic patient receives a hand-written prayer letter at the conclusion of their visit.

In August 2022, I joined the organization as Director of Clinical Services and was the clinic's first on-staff clinical pharmacist. Beyond my duties of managing the clinical operations, I began taking consultations with patients to assist in managing their disease states, laboratory values, and medications. While many of my interactions with patients happened in-person, I often followed up with some of my most medically fragile patients with phone calls to facilitate closer monitoring of their disease states. In 2024, one particular patient was desperate to gain control of his newly diagnosed diabetes. Little did I know at the time that this patient would impact the way I approached my practice moving forward.

DOI: 10.37573/9781585287727.016

This 28-year-old African male arrived at the clinic after being in the hospital the previous week due to polyuria (large volume of urine), polydipsia (excessive thirst), vomiting, weight loss, and an elevated blood glucose of around 800 mg/dL. His hemoglobin A1C, a test to monitor diabetes, was high at 11.5%. The hospital physician had diagnosed the patient with new-onset diabetes, noting that he suspected underlying type 1 diabetes mellitus. The patient did not have medical insurance, so more specific diagnostic tests were limited at that point in his care. As he completed the check-in forms before his appointment with the nurse practitioner, he appeared anxious. During his appointment, he expressed confusion about his diagnosis and voiced concerns about his insulin dosing. At this point, the nurse practitioner asked me to assist with his care.

After much discussion and some basic laboratory tests, we landed on a treatment plan for the patient as well as a plan for follow-up. It was determined that I would provide close follow-up via scheduled phone calls to monitor the patient's glucose levels, with the primary goal of keeping him out of the hospital. At the end of this appointment, the patient relayed that he felt more comfortable knowing that he would finally receive help in these first few weeks of his diagnosis. As is offered to all our patients, he accepted prayer from our nurse practitioner prior to leaving the exam room, and he humbly received the hand-written prayer letter upon checking out. At the conclusion of his visit, I finished my chart notes, reviewing his intake form, which had been uploaded in the "Documents" section of his chart, one more time. Among the information asked on the intake form is a "Religious Preference" section. The patient had left this section blank.

Over the next 3 days, I connected with the patient daily as planned. He seemed motivated to get his blood sugar levels under control and to learn about his diabetes. There was a slight challenge in communication, as English was the patient's second language; however, he always demonstrated that he understood and promised to adhere to all treatment changes. On the third day of follow-up calls, I could sense he seemed more anxious and disheartened. His glucose readings continued to be severely elevated, and he expressed fear and concern surrounding his diagnosis. He tearfully asked me if he would have to stay on insulin forever, and he expressed confusion as to why this was happening to him. He quickly followed these concerns with a question that would open a new line of trust between us and extend a new level of care. With a sort of desperation in his voice, he asked, "Are you Christian? Will you keep me in your prayers?"

In that moment, I realized I had not been consistent in asking my patients about their spiritual care needs. While it was common practice in clinic, I had never truly prioritized this practice during my follow-up phone calls. Without hesitation, I told the patient that, of course, I would keep him in my prayers, but then I asked him if I could pray for him "right now" over the phone. The sense of relief that emanated from the patient's voice as he responded, "Yes, please! Yes, please!" touched me deeply. I began to pray for him: for peace and understanding, for strength and perseverance, for support from his family and friends, for blessings in his life and for his family, and for complete healing if it is God's will. During the entire time, I could hear my patient quietly praying with me in his native language, seemingly in agreement with my words. It was an emotional moment—one full of hope, surrender, connectedness, and trust. At the end of the prayer, the patient was again tearful, but his voice expressed gratitude and optimism instead of fear and worry as he repeated "Thank you, thank you" over and over. We had not only ended the call with a revised plan for his insulin, but a renewed sense of trust in the healthcare process and a space for spirituality in his healing.

This patient was only with our clinic for a month before his insurance application was approved and he transitioned to another clinic, but in that short time frame, I had the opportunity to interact with him 12 additional times. I remember our phone call the very next day; he called our clinic before I even had the chance to reach out to him. He seemed much more optimistic and determined to face his diabetes diagnosis. With each call, he entrusted me with additional insights into his life and struggles, and with each day that passed, his glucose readings improved. We also made sure to end every conversation in prayer. At his last appointment, tears streamed down his face because he did not want to leave the clinic's care. He voiced concern that his new doctor wouldn't provide the same level of support and that he felt "seen and heard" at our clinic. Moreover, he expressed that "they won't pray with me like you do."

To ease his concerns, I made a call directly to his new doctor to make his transition of care as smooth as possible, highlighting his current plan of care as well as his desire for additional diabetes education, closer follow-up, and the importance of prayer to him. Additionally, I told the patient that he was always welcome to call the clinic or stop by if he needed prayer. Our patient left grateful, and 4 months later he showed up at our clinic, informing us that his A1C was down to 6.5% and that he no longer needed insulin according to his doctor. He donated all his unopened insulin pens to our clinic.

This patient and these interactions helped shape the way that I approached other patients moving forward. I began to prioritize being more consistent in offering prayer and in asking about spiritual needs, not just physical, mental, and emotional. Just as I had experienced with this patient, I continue to discover that this opens doors with other patients to be more trusting, more dedicated to their health, and more likely to follow up. I believe that holistic care doesn't stop at the physical, mental, emotional, and social, but healthcare professionals are often not encouraged or supported in addressing the spiritual needs. Sometimes, the missing piece to a patient's medical success isn't a better or different medication. Sometimes, the missing piece is filling the gap of spiritual yearning in a patient's overall well-being.

Providence and Presence

James T. Miller

PharmD, BCCCP

When pharmacy students and residents get their first experiences rounding with a large, academic, multidisciplinary intensive care unit (ICU) team, they often tell me, "I feel like I'm not doing anything." They aren't accustomed to the patient population, the disease states that bring patients to our unit, or the primary literature in the area, so it's entirely natural that they feel unequipped for what I'm asking of them. Much of that confidence and sense of belonging comes with repeated exposure and experience, but I encourage them in the same way I encourage myself: "You have to be there for the little things, so that you're there and trusted for the big things."

Life as an ICU pharmacist includes lots of small things, such as adjusting medication doses, assessing the potential for drug–drug interactions, and ensuring the compatibility of infusions, but it also includes unpredictable moments where your skills and knowledge are at once pushed and stretched to their utmost. In order to be effective and reliable in those less frequently occurring but awash-in-adrenaline moments, we have to hone our practice in the more mundane.

In the ICU, it's easy to take for granted the position in which we find ourselves, the responsibility that we've been granted, and the gravity of the environment. We show up every day and do largely similar things as the day before, but for patients and their families, it's often the worst day of their lives. While we grumble about the state of employee parking, others are suffocating under the harrowing and heavy blanket of fear and grief for their loved ones. Clinicians keep showing up to do the things that diminish in significance over time in our own eyes, because we do them so often, but those "diminished" things hold tremendous importance to the patients and families who find themselves in such unfamiliar and frightening territory. As pharmacists, we underestimate the value of just being there and caring.

I didn't initially set out to incorporate my faith into my professional practice. It's not always clear whether to, how to, or if it's even welcome. But when a dear friend from high school was admitted to our ICU for complications of leukemia, and I saw her parents' faces on rounds, how could I not sit with them after the team moved to the next patient? We went to a high school dance together. Her parents fed me at their home. If I've sat at your dinner table, I can sit at your bedside. Being *only* a professional in this moment didn't seem to be an option. All *I* did was come to work that day, but providence gave them a friendly and familiar face.

Years later, a member of our church was admitted to another ICU, and I was one flight of stairs away. We had studied the Bible together, sung together, and

DOI: 10.37573/9781585287727.017

prayed together. It wouldn't be weird to visit him and his wife and pray with them; it would be weird not to. I was there, they knew me well, and it seemed a small thing to me, but it wasn't a small thing to them.

"Love your neighbor as yourself" (Matthew 22:39, English Standard Version [ESV]) is half of the greatest commandment to a Christian but is widely understood to be a wise proverb or at least a good idea by many others.[1] When my literal neighbor had surgery and needed a few days to recover in the ICU, I found myself at his bedside, too. I still have the picture his wife took of our team while we were rounding. She was so glad (and proud) to see her neighbor, half her age, as part of her husband's care team and talks about it to this day, although her husband has since passed. Our proximity in the ICU *and* in the neighborhood has bound us together in a way neither of us will forget. To this day, she still joins our family for celebrations of holidays and birthdays. I can think of a handful of other people who I either knew well or knew well enough to stop in and say hello when they were in the hospital. They don't expect much, or anything, really, and I may not have hours to give. But nobody thinks I will anyway. There is a ministry of presence. Before Job's friends lost the plot, they sat with their bereft friend for 7 days before speaking a single word. Sometimes the sick need a word, and sometimes they just need someone who cares about them to sit with them.

A number of years ago, the ICU I work in participated in a clinical trial called the ICU Liberation Study.[2] It assessed the clinical benefits of a bundle of interventions summarized by the acronym, ABCDEF. The "F" stands for "Family Engagement and Empowerment." It's often true that nobody knows a patient like their family. One of the most interesting and hopeful results of the trial was that not only did the bundle improve outcomes, but every component of it did the same, independent of the others. Family presence helps ICU patients do better. I've developed a corollary theory on why the bundle works: the more normal you can make an ICU patient feel, the better they do. There's only one "F" in the bundle, but friends with familiar faces are Fs, too.

I do believe in God's providence. Merriam-Webster defines it as "divine guidance or care."[3] My own definition of it is His active sovereignty, meaning that He's in control of everything and isn't sitting back watching our stories unfold. I believe that God has put me where I am and given me the skills and knowledge to do what I do. I still hit the snooze button too many times, and I still look forward to going home at the end of the workday, but I don't think it's an accident that I go where I go every day, and I don't think it's an accident that you go where you go. In the seemingly small act of getting up and going to work day after day, we have the opportunity to minister to people who don't think what we're doing is mundane. Your presence is a ministry to others.[3] They remember who visited them when they were sick. They remember who held their hand when they were scared. They remember who prayed for their healing and for their peace when they were losing hope.

Going to work again tomorrow can make you feel like a pharmacy student going to ICU rounds, believing that you're not really doing anything. At least not anything of importance, we tell our impostor syndrome-suffering selves. But that's not the way other people see you: sick patients who you help don't see you and your work that way. They're immensely grateful. They don't even know how to repay you, so they bring in donuts for the unit.

Direct patient care may not be part of your job responsibilities—no matter. If you work with other people, you will not find yourself lacking the opportunity to sit, to listen, to encourage, to build up, and to strengthen. Showing up, repeatedly, scorning whatever mundanity it brings ministers to many. *Not* showing up deprives them of your unique talents, skills, knowledge, and love.[3] It's just another day on the grind for you, but not for them. In the words of the teacher, Solomon, "*I perceived that there is nothing better for them than to be joyful and to do good as long as they live; also, that everyone should eat and drink and take pleasure in all his toil—this is God's gift to man*" (Ecclesiastes 3:11-12).[1] By virtue of your relationships in the community combined with your professional proximity to and presence among the sick, you have great opportunity to bring peace and rest where it is desperately needed. It may seem a small thing, even inconsequential in your eyes, but the pebbles you throw make ripples that the sick and suffering see as healing waves.

References

1. *The ESV Study Bible: English Standard Version*. Wheaton, IL: Crossway; 2008.
2. Pun B, Balas MC, Barnes-Daly M, et al. Caring for critically ill patients with the ABCDEF bundle: results of the ICU Liberation Collaborative in over 15,000 adults. *Crit Care Med.* 2019;47(1):3-14. https://doi.org/10.1097/CCM.0000000000003482
3. Noble A. *On getting out of bed: The burden and gift of living.* Downers Grove, IL: IVP; 2023.

Presence as Medicine: A Story of Unborn, Spirit, and Trust in Patient Care

Phuoc Anne Nguyen
PharmD, MS, BCPS, FTSHP

It was a gray morning, rain gently draping the hospital in quiet stillness. The hum of infusion pumps and the soft shuffle of footsteps filled the space. That was when I met Mrs. T. She sat in a recliner by the window, gazing at the sky as if waiting for it to change. At 79, she carried a serene grace—a floral shawl over her shoulders, silver hair neatly tied. There was dignity in her stillness, reminding me of my own mother—gentle, wise, and composed. She had been hospitalized for a gram-negative bacteremia and was preparing for discharge with plans for home IV antibiotic therapy. I visited her in my role as a transitions-of-care pharmacist, reviewing her medications and ensuring a safe plan for treatment at home.

I greeted her softly: "Good morning. My name is Anne, your pharmacist. I'm here to go over the medications you'll be taking at home."

She offered a tired yet polite smile. "Thank you. I suppose we'll be talking about those antibiotics again."

We reviewed the treatment plan, the side effects, timing, and home infusion logistics. Everything was in order; yet her voice carried a quiet heaviness, something not documented in her medical record. I asked gently, "Mrs. T, is there something on your mind today? You seem a bit distant."

She sighed. "It's just lonely here. My daughters both work. They call every night, but no one can visit during the day. I feel . . . not myself when I'm in the hospital."

Just then, a chaplain knocked softly and asked, "Would you like me to pray with you?"

Mrs. T. smiled kindly but shook her head. "I'm Buddhist. I prefer to meditate."

The chaplain nodded respectfully and stepped out. I stayed.

"I meditate too," I said.

Her eyes lit up in surprise. "Really?"

"I practice Awakened Stillness Meditation under the guidance of Awakened Zen Master Thich Dieu Thien, the founder of Universal Door Meditation Center here in Houston," I shared. "I found her during a time of deep inner struggle. Since her enlightenment in 2001, she has guided countless people of all faiths and

DOI: 10.37573/9781585287727.018

backgrounds to return to the Unborn Source, freeing themselves from the "born mind" that causes suffering, to truly live with peace and freedom. Her teachings changed my life."

She asked, "The Unborn . . . what does that mean?"

I replied, "It is the original, pure mind—open and bright, free from thought, ego, and suffering."

I invited her to practice Awakened Stillness Meditation with me. We sat quietly together, breathing in and breathing out, allowing the mind to settle, not following thoughts, just noticing the awareness that observes them. After about 10 minutes, her face softened, her eyes brightened, and a natural smile appeared—calm, genuine, serene.

I smiled and said, "The Unborn Mind doesn't need a prescription. It's always within us." She chuckled softly: "Exactly."

I noticed her phone nearby. "Do you have a chant you like to listen to?"

"The Heart Sutra," she said. "It brings me peace, especially at night."

"Would you like to hear it now?"

She nodded. I opened YouTube, found Awakened Zen Master Thich Dieu Thien's chanting of the Heart Sutra and placed the phone beside her. The sacred sound flowed gently into the room . . . deep, soothing, alive. The hospital room seemed to shift; warmer and more luminous, it was as if the room, too, was breathing.

We sat in silence, two human beings, two breaths in rhythm with the chant. Five minutes passed. The hum of the IV pump faded; the fluorescent lights softened behind closed eyes. In that stillness, the hospital room transformed into a small temple of the soul.

When we opened our eyes, hers shimmered. "For a moment," she whispered, "I forgot I was in the hospital. I felt . . . home."

"Your mind was home," I said. "Inside yourself."

Before leaving, I documented not only her medication plan but also what mattered most—her Buddhist meditation practice, her need for stillness, and quiet infusion times. I spoke with the nursing staff to help create that sacred space, not just clinical care, but whole-person care: body, mind, and Unborn Spirit.

Before I left, she reached for my hand.

"You helped me see who I truly am," she said softly. "Not a busy mind, not just a body with IV lines, but a Pure Mind . . . walking the path of awakening. You saw me," she added. "Not just my illness."

And at that moment, I understood—presence itself is the deepest medicine. Healing is not only in what we do, but in how we show up—fully, sincerely, and with pure awareness. Amid medication lists and lab results, let us not forget the sacred stillness between two breaths, where science meets the Unborn Mind, and where care becomes connection.

Let us honor every expression of that Unborn Stillness within our hospitals: a soft chant in the corner, a prayer before dawn, or a silent moment of returning within. These are not interruptions; they are part of healing itself.

Let us ask our patients, "What brings you peace?" and pause long enough to truly listen. Because sometimes, healing does not begin with a prescription but with a return to the Unborn Mind.

Breath by breath.

Heart to heart.

That is where we meet.

Amazing Grace

Agatha Nolen
PhD, MDiv, FASHP

When I started at a new health system as the Director of Pharmacy, I didn't just want to learn the job; I wanted to know the people. So, I met with every pharmacy staff member one-on-one, and I also sat down with the other department directors to start building those relationships. A few weeks into my new job, I met with the Director of Rehabilitation, who mentioned that he played the guitar occasionally during his Sunday church services. We had a good discussion about how our churches use music in our worship services—me as a Roman Catholic and him as a Southern Baptist. He shared his desire to conduct a weekly sing-along with his rehabilitation (rehab) patients. These were primarily older patients who had limited mobility following a stroke, and he was eager to provide activities that would help them get out of their rooms and socialize in a group setting.

The following month, while I was meeting with the Director of Respiratory Therapy, he mentioned that he sang in his church choir, and an idea began to form! The three of us decided to try a sing-along with patients and staff the following Wednesday afternoon in the common space of the rehab unit. We had a guitar player and three voices; we just needed to choose some music. We photocopied 10 well-worn hymns that we hoped would be universally known and prepared 30 booklets for the staff, patients, and their caregivers to use during the activity. We had planned to practice the day before, but like most hospital days, higher priority tasks popped up that prevented a rehearsal. So, we decided to "do our best" for our first session.

Wednesday came and we assembled at 1 p.m. in the common space of the rehab unit, waiting for our patients to arrive. Slowly they came, with most in wheelchairs accompanied by a caregiver. At 1:30 p.m., we passed out the hymn booklets and invited everyone to join us in song. For the first few songs, no one joined us, and the three of us sang in harmony with the guitar accompaniment. Then, we heard a few faint voices from staff members, patients, and some caregivers who cautiously joined in.

One patient was an octogenarian who had suffered a stroke and had been confined to bed for months. She sat strapped into her wheelchair, slumped and motionless, with a caregiver at her side. There was no sign that she was aware of her surroundings—or even that she knew she had been brought into the common space of the rehab unit. The Director of Rehabilitation gently reminded us that many of

DOI: 10.37573/9781585287727.019

the patients might not respond to our sing-along, yet it was still important—and good for them—to be brought out of their rooms for a change of environment.

We gathered confidence in our singing and playing (even without a practice session)! On the eighth song, a transformation occurred. As we began to belt out *Amazing Grace*, our octogenarian sat up straight in her wheelchair and began singing. She wasn't even looking at our hymn book! She knew all four verses and sang each one perfectly in tune! After we sang the last note and started on hymn number nine, she slipped back into her slumped position in her wheelchair and sang no more.

The three of us remember our teary finish, knowing that the hymn had awakened something deep inside of her that we were unable to reach otherwise. It had a profound effect on us, and we considered how haphazardly we had thrown our group together, wanting to sing as much for ourselves as for the patients.

We continued to hold sing-alongs every Wednesday for 4 months, perfecting our harmony and adding a piano part on select songs. It became the time of the week that I looked forward to the most, an opportunity to decompress from the pressures of patient care and endless clinical challenges. A time to just rest with a song in our heart, knowing that our music was reaching into an unknown realm. These times of singing changed me. I realized that we can never truly know what someone is going through or what might reach their heart, but even so, we keep trying, bringing moments of joy and comfort whenever and wherever we can.

We were not at all surprised that every Wednesday the same scene would repeat itself. We would sing to a roomful of patients and caregivers with different levels of participation. Each week, our favorite patient would sit, slumped and unresponsive in her wheelchair, until we started to sing *Amazing Grace*. Each week she would awaken, sing all the verses with us, and then fall back into a peaceful sleep until the next time.

Over the years, I've met a few churchgoers who have shared how much they dislike the song *Amazing Grace*, saying that it is "overused" or "too easy to sing." It has been criticized because out of the 150 words in the original six verses, only 21 have more than one syllable. To those who are critical of the song, I say, "Let me tell you a story. . . ."

My story in that rehab unit occurred three decades ago; more recently, President Barack Obama sang *Amazing Grace* at the funeral for South Carolina State Senator Reverend Clementa Pinckney, who was killed along with eight others while leading a Bible study at his church in Charleston, SC, in June 2015. The song continues to comfort and inspire throughout the generations.

My spiritual activities have been important to me in my overall work as a pharmacist, because my faith has never been separate from the roles that I've had as a pharmacist. Whether it was working in a free clinic, in an intensive care unit or operating room satellite pharmacy, or as a pharmacy administrator, I tried to approach everyone as someone who bears God's image. It might have been a patient, coworker, nurse, physician, or family member, but I hope that I treated them with the dignity and respect that they deserved in every interaction. I also recognized early in my career that some encounters are easier than others, and we often don't know how our actions impact people. We must trust that how we treat others makes a difference in their lives and in ours.

A Whisper Before the Injection: A Lesson in Spiritual Presence

Alvena Noor

PharmD candidate

I am a student pharmacist and have recently begun exploring the deeper, human dimensions of patient care, including the essential but often overlooked role of spirituality.

In pharmacy school, we learn about drug interactions, contraindications, and lab work. During my first year as a PharmD student, I was just beginning to grasp the interconnected concepts of drug mechanisms, pharmacokinetics, and patient counseling. Still, no class truly prepares you for the thick silence in someone's eyes when they are truly terrified—or for the solace they find in a whispered prayer. This was indeed a revelation for me. I now know that healing is about vanquishing disease and also about deep respect, presence, and faith. The most important lesson that I absorbed after enrolling in pharmacy school was not from the books I read or lectures I attended, but from an understated moment during my clinical shadowing.

In my first semester, I had the opportunity to shadow pharmacists at a university-affiliated teaching hospital. The hospital endured a continuous pulse of life—the lulling monotony of beeping monitors, hurried footsteps, and sterile scents of room temperature antiseptic. As much as I had seen hospitals portrayed in movies, I had never set foot in one. I was deeply anxious while walking through the corridors, not having the faintest idea about what I might observe or if I would be able to contribute to any patient's care. Clutching my clipboard, I was prepared to jot down doses and interactions, taking notes as if I were in a classroom. It was not the prescriptions noted that lingered with me, but rather the stillness I encountered. It was breathtaking as I looked into my patient's eyes and saw a representative of all of humankind who was very still and deeply spiritual. I learned a profound lesson in that moment, realizing that healing went beyond controlling blood sugar levels or lowering high blood pressure. Healing involved enabling patients to bring their entire selves to the experience of care, including their faith. My patient was asking for care far deeper than any text could impart; she was asking for my presence.

It was an ordinary afternoon in the general ward. I had been assigned to a 68-year-old woman with type II diabetes. During rounds, I could not help but notice her trembling hands as she balanced an insulin syringe. She narrowed her eyes each time a nurse uttered the word "insulin."

DOI: 10.37573/9781585287727.020

As a student observer, the patient safety protocols prohibited me from giving medications, which freed me to concentrate on observing my patients. I stood at her bedside as a nurse was preparing a subcutaneous insulin injection. At that moment, the patient turned her body to her right and slowly reached under her pillow, retrieving a small *tasbeeh* (prayer beads). She gripped it tightly and whispered something, perhaps "*Bismillah*." *Bismillah* is Arabic and means "in the name of God." It is an Islamic phrase frequently recited by Muslims before performing daily activities and religious practices, including prayer and any task where you wish to have success and protection from harm.

The nurse took a deep breath and asked gently, "Would you like to pray?"

The patient nodded. "Just one minute, let me ask Allah for ease. I feel scared every time."

The nurse smiled, stepped back, and waited. I remained quiet, and at that moment, I was touched. The nurse was unhurried, not irritated that she was delayed in caring for her next patient, but instead, she was fully focused on this patient and her needs. The patient was not only actively receiving care but also integrating her faith into it. Receiving an insulin injection was not just a clinical act for her but a moment of spiritual surrender.

I approached the nurse later and asked, "Does this happen often?"

"All the time," she replied. "Some patients pray, some ask for a call to the masjid (mosque), and some even cry for forgiveness. Their bodies may be in our hands, but their hearts are with God."

I will always remember that statement: "Their bodies may be in our hands, but their hearts are with God."

The next day, I accompanied the clinical pharmacist as she reviewed the medication profile with the patient. I gently asked the patient if she felt okay with her treatment. She said, "My child, the medicines help, but it is the remembrance of Allah that gives me strength. If someone reminds me of Him during these times, then I am less alone."

As the nurse was preparing the next dose of insulin, I gently said, "Say *Bismillah*, Aunty." Her smile told me that we had connected. Her shoulders relaxed as the tension in her body was released.

I didn't perform a medical procedure, nor provide any medication reconciliation or counseling, but something shifted. At that moment, I realized that spiritual care does not always require elaborate plans. It's simply the act of witnessing someone's faith and participating in that space with them. It may be a single word, but I was able to offer presence and encourage her to utter "*Bismillah*." With her, I did not pray. I did not give scriptural quotes. What I did was honor her way of relating to the Divine in a hospital ward that was sterile, bright with fluorescent lights, and filled with needles and charts.

This patient served as my lens to glimpse the meaning of whole-person care. She was not merely a patient with high blood sugar. She was a woman of faith with a soul trying to find solace from the storm of illness that surrounded her.

Ever since that day, I have been more observant during my hospital rounds. A rosary tied to bed rails, whispered Quranic verses, and patients requesting to postpone medications until after prayers. These do not constitute a disruption; they connect as sacred pauses. Acknowledging these does not step us out of our professional boundaries. It is part of our personhood as pharmacists in training. I've also become more empathetic not only to Muslims but to patients who seek meaning during illness. Illness strips people of control. Faith in a spiritual power often restores it.

What I learned from this patient wasn't how to dose insulin. I learned how to dose "presence."

This impacted my relationship with the patient through the simple acknowledgment of her spiritual need, and I was able to form a bond even as an observer. This changed the interaction from a clinical one to a more kindhearted and human one. My patient became more at ease, compliant, and trusting, because I regarded her as a person rather than a diabetes case file. The bridge connecting the scientific and the soulful was built with that single word, "*Bismillah*."

If I were asked to give advice to practitioners who want to incorporate more spiritual care into their practice as pharmacy professionals, it would be three simple actions: create space, observe, and listen. You do not need to have all the answers. To start, silence is required. Provide space for prayer or fasting. Display reverence for all symbols and sacred rituals. Regarding spirituality as irrelevant to a patient's care is the worst approach to take. Whole-person care does not call for preaching, but presence, which starts with modesty and humility.

Honoring Faith in the Pharmacy Setting: Spiritual Encounters in Community Care

Sue Paul
RPh

I have practiced pharmacy for more than 30 years and for the past 10 years primarily in ambulatory care where I enjoy helping patients reduce medication burden by eliminating duplicate or unnecessary therapy through diet, lifestyle education, and addressing social determinants of health. I often assist with finding cost-effective alternatives of care. But it is working as a clinical pharmacist in two urban Federally Qualified Health Centers (FQHCs) in a large Ohio city that has offered me a front-row seat to view the raw and often challenging realities of people's lives. These clinics serve some of the most underserved populations in our community, including individuals facing chronic illness, homelessness, addiction, trauma, and poverty. It is in this environment, amidst the heartache and healing, that I have discovered how addressing patients' spiritual needs can be just as vital as discussing medication regimens or lifestyle changes. My practice setting allows me to engage with patients on a regular basis with up to 15 encounters per day. Addressing patients' spiritual needs is not always part of my patient visits; it is only when I feel prompted by an unexplained nudge.

I remember one encounter vividly. A woman in her late 50s came to my clinic for a follow-up after being started on medication for uncontrolled diabetes and depression. I reviewed her A1C level with her and noted that her diabetes was improving slightly, but her demeanor was not. She sat quietly in the exam room, eyes downcast, her responses clipped. As we reviewed her medication, I was surprised that she mentioned she was no longer taking her antidepressant. She didn't feel that it was helpful and was experiencing side effects.

Her eyes welled with tears. She finally spoke, "It's just hard. I feel like I'm trying and nothing gets better. I pray, but I don't think God is listening to me anymore."

It wasn't the first time a patient had mentioned their faith while discussing their health. I have learned that when patients bring up spiritual matters, it's often a tender opening. In that moment, I had an invitation to continue the conversation.

"Can I ask you something? Do you have a faith you can lean into?"

She nodded, "I used to go to church, and I do believe in Jesus. I just feel . . . forgotten."

DOI: 10.37573/9781585287727.021

I reached into my pocket and asked if I could offer her a "little Jesus."

She shook her head, "Yes," and I held out a tiny plastic figurine of Jesus, no bigger than an inch tall. It's something I keep with me intentionally, knowing that moments like this may arise.

"I know it's small, but sometimes it helps to have something tangible—a reminder that you're not alone. That He's still here, even if He feels quiet."

She stared at the figurine for a long moment before reaching out to take it, her hands trembling. "Thank you," she whispered with tears in her eyes.

That brief exchange—barely 3 minutes—shifted the tone of our relationship entirely. From that day forward, she greeted me with warmth and would mention that she still has her "little Jesus." She became more consistent with her follow-up appointments and began to take her medications regularly, including her antidepressants. Her health has improved, yes—but more than that, her hope seems to have been restored.

Another patient at my other FQHC was an older gentleman recovering from a recent stroke. He had been despondent and uncooperative with his treatment plan, and his provider asked if I would talk with him about medication adherence. After a few minutes of discussion, I asked him to tell me what brings him joy. He mentioned music and Jesus, and he shared that he hadn't played his guitar lately since his stroke; he even used to be in a band. I suggested that he check his blood pressure before and after playing his guitar and to write the numbers of his blood pressure down. We were able to give him a blood pressure monitor and educate him on the proper technique for monitoring his own blood pressure. Since he had mentioned Jesus, I also gave him a "little Jesus" figure. That led us to a rich, meaningful conversation about strength, suffering, and healing. Over the next few office visits, he confidently started following our treatment plans with enthusiasm, not because of a new medication, but because someone saw and encouraged him in his joyful habits and honored his spiritual practices.

The lessons I've learned from these encounters are numerous. First, spiritual needs are not separate from physical or emotional health; they are interwoven. When people are suffering, the ache goes beyond the body. A patient can be physically stable but spiritually despondent—and if we miss that layer, we miss an opportunity to offer whole-person care. Second, I've learned the importance of discernment. Not every patient wants to talk about spiritual matters. But many do, and they're just waiting for someone to ask. At our health centers, patients complete a social history intake form, which includes a question about religious affiliation. I glance at this section when I feel prompted. If a patient identifies as Christian, Jewish, Muslim, or "spiritual but not religious," it gives me context and language I can use respectfully when the moment arises.

Most of the spiritual conversations that I have are initiated organically. I might notice a patient struggling with grief, shame, or fear and ask gently if they have a faith that they can lean into. If they mention Jesus or identify as Christian, I'll ask if I can offer them a "little Jesus" and give them the small Jesus figurine with the conversation unfolding from there. It's a quiet, nonthreatening gesture, but it opens a door. Once that door is opened, many patients feel seen and safe in a new way. I offer to pray to God with patients even though they may not acknowledge being a Christian.

Of course, not every spiritual conversation yields immediate visible results, but that's not the point. I don't initiate these conversations to convert or counsel. I see them as part of recognizing the fullness of who my patients are. Faith, for many, is central to identity and healing. Acknowledging that is simply good, compassionate care.

Personally, my own faith informs my willingness to engage. Prior to each appointment, I say a quick prayer to the Holy Spirit for wisdom. I don't force or preach, but I also don't hide what motivates my work. I believe every patient is made in God's image and that brings dignity to every interaction. I've seen time and time again how reminding someone of their spiritual resources can rekindle hope, improve engagement with care, and create a bridge of trust between provider and patient.

Ultimately, working in these FQHCs has taught me that spiritual care doesn't have to be elaborate. It can be a question. A pause. A tiny figurine. A willingness to listen. These small things, done in love, matter deeply.

The Healing Power of Prayer

Susan L. Ravnan
PharmD, FCSHP

I have been a pharmacist for more than 30 years in an academic environment with patient care practice settings ranging from inpatient hospital, critical care, internal medicine, outpatient retail, and independent community practice to ambulatory care. My current practice setting is an ambulatory care telehealth service, focusing on acute ambulatory care problems. Until this year, I have never considered the spiritual needs of my patients, despite recognizing the importance of spirituality in my own life for many years.

The notion of patient-centered, whole-person or holistic care, defined as caring for a patient's physical, emotional, mental, social, and spiritual well-being, is not new to the 21st century. During each decade, one aspect of holistic care has been weighed above another, but spiritual care has never fully been adopted into this approach, and this has been true of my practice as well.

If I considered spirituality and more specifically, the power of prayer, a fundamental aspect of my overall well-being, why did I not address this with my patients? The answer is summed up simply as fear. Fear of offending a patient who may be of a different religion, fear of losing my job, fear of not having enough time, and fear of being seen as proselytizing someone in a vulnerable position. This year, prayer became an essential aspect in my practice. I would like to share my experience with three patients, with diverse spiritual backgrounds, in which I offered prayer as a means of practicing whole-person care. It is my hope that through this essay, others will find personal ways to include spiritual care in their practice as well.

Through my 30-minute telehealth phone conversation with patients, I often identify aspects of the patient's spiritual/religious needs. After introducing myself to each patient and explaining the reason for the call, I always ask them, "How are you doing today?" Through the tone of their voice, three patients each displayed a general sense of uneasiness or angst about their life. I merely offered a listening ear, not worrying that I only had 30 minutes to talk about the "real" reason for my call. After speaking freely about their lives in general, patient #1 offered that she was a devout Christian with a strong social network within her church who was praying for her and that her religious mechanism provides a way of managing life's challenges. Patient #2 did not consider herself as a religious/spiritual person. Patient #3 stated that she knew of Jesus but did not have a personal relationship with God. I asked patients #2 and #3 if they had anyone or anything to help them manage the

DOI: 10.37573/9781585287727.022

stresses of life. They both suggested that religion/spirituality was a way to cope with stress and offered personal information about their spirituality and connection to a religious institution. The patients offered this information voluntarily; I did not ask specifically about their religious or spiritual beliefs, but I was willing to listen to their answers to some of my general questions.

The spiritual information that they provided at this time guided me further. I proceeded to discuss the reason for my call and addressed their physical condition and how medication would contribute to better well-being. Addressing their spiritual aspect was individualized. For patient #1, I asked if she would like me to pray with her over the phone, and she agreed. She thanked me for the prayers and expressed appreciation that I had recognized and addressed her nonphysical needs. For patient #2, I acknowledged to her that I realized she was not religious, but explained that I was, and that I would pray for her and check in with her at our next encounter if she was agreeable. She was appreciative and thanked me, too. With patient #3, I asked if she would like me to pray that God would personally be revealed to her. She too welcomed my prayers.

At the closing of each conversation, the tone of their voices softened. I presumed that my recognition of their spiritual needs went beyond healing of their physical or mental needs. For patient #1, it was significant, as if her burdens had never existed. For patients #2 and #3, the change was not as significant but still noticeable. However, after the second encounter with these patients, the tone became significantly different. The patient sounded more optimistic. I did not share with the two patients that I had been praying for them over the past month, but I did call to follow up to see how they were doing and how they were tolerating the new medication prescribed during the previous encounter.

Did my spiritual conversations improve the patient–provider relationship? Were they more apt to follow my medication advice knowing that I provided a more holistic patient care approach? I am not sure, but I do believe that they were more comfortable being honest with me about their wishes regarding their personal healthcare needs without fear.

The impact of prayer for my patients on my life cannot be overlooked. Life and the practice of pharmacy provide many opportunities for stress and anxiety to emerge in my life. However, I am always astonished by how praying for my patients can calm my spirit as well. The main reason I entered pharmacy was to improve the health of my patients. I am grateful for the positive outcomes that medications can provide for physical ailments. However, there is a state of calmness that is present during our health challenges that can only be achieved through spiritual care. It transcends all human understanding as explainable by modern science.

I want to encourage others to begin looking for ways to practice whole-person care by identifying and meeting the spiritual needs of the patient along with their physical and mental needs. One simple step is to listen to your patient. Let the patient guide the conversation but be ready to engage with the patient and their spiritual needs. This interaction should never be driven by a protocol. This is about one patient and one pharmacist working together to improve the patient's comfort and well-being in all three realms of their personal identity: the physical, mental, and spiritual.

Cura Personalis in the Dominican Republic

Edward M. Saito
PharmD, BCACP, DPLA

In 2011, I had the privilege of living with and serving individuals in the Dominican Republic while on an advanced pharmacy practice experience (APPE) rotation sponsored by the college of pharmacy that I attended. This program was a multidisciplinary, cultural immersion experience that promoted and fostered genuine encounters with rural residents of the Dominican Republic while providing basic healthcare services and education. Participants live with host families for 3 to 4 weeks, working in a small medical or dental clinic in the morning and providing educational talks or "*charlas*" (a chat or conversation) to the community in the afternoon. This experience was grounded in Ignatian spirituality, which emphasizes the values of *cura personalis* (care for the "whole person"). Through these values, participants are invited to foster a spirit of service to the Dominicans that recognizes the physical, emotional, and spiritual needs of each person.

International service trips are often viewed as opportunities to provide charity care to underserved individuals and to gain better insight into the causes and experience of global poverty. However, this program focuses on the transformation of the volunteers as they connect with others through relationship and service. Indeed, Pope Francis, in his encyclical letter, *Fratelli Tutti: On Fraternity and Social Friendship,* says that we must build a "culture of encounter" to accompany others who are suffering and that "the process of building fraternity, be it local or universal, can only be undertaken by spirits that are free and open to authentic encounters."[1] To truly care for the whole person requires that we acknowledge and address the spiritual needs of our patients alongside their physical health concerns. For example, providing a 30-day supply of hydrochlorothiazide could improve high blood pressure, but to provide effective and enduring care to our Dominican host communities, we first had to understand and appreciate the full cultural and religious context in which we were working. We did more than just dispense medication; we gained deeper insight into the social and spiritual needs of our patients whose culture was different from our own.

One weekend, a small group of pharmacy, medical, and nursing students were invited to visit an elderly woman who lived alone on the outskirts of the community. Because it was physically challenging for her to come to our morning clinic in town, we walked for 30 minutes along an unpaved path through dense forest to

DOI: 10.37573/9781585287727.023

arrive at her home. We spent the afternoon conducting a basic health evaluation and visiting with her while she offered coffee and snacks. At one point, she asked to go to her bedroom to lay down for a few minutes due to the onset of a headache. When we heard her cry out in agony, we rushed in to find her rigid and convulsing. After a quick evaluation, we determined that she needed to be examined by our attending physician who was still in town. We spent several hours carrying the woman back to town in a chair, and after evaluation by our physician, she was transported to a medical facility in the nearest city. We later learned that she had suffered a severe stroke and later died. Our group of volunteers was devastated and in shock, left to debrief what had happened. The tragedy of her passing was made even more poignant by the cultural distance between us. As Americans, we were with her when she suffered her attack, yet we could not offer the familiar presence, language, or customs that might have brought her comfort in that moment. Instead, we bore witness as outsiders, feeling both the weight of her loss and the limits of what we could give.

How could we possibly continue with our daily work of providing healthcare to this community amid this tragedy? It could have been viewed as insensitive if we carried on as if nothing had happened, and yet we were only there for a limited time to fulfill our program objectives. The parish priest who provided spiritual counseling for members of the local community, and who was part of our group, helped us to process the loss.

We learned that a key element of Catholic culture in the Dominican Republic involves a 9-day period of mourning following a person's death: "*los nueve dias*." This practice is a structured way for the family and community to process the grief. So, with humility, we asked the community if we could participate in the family's *novena*, 9 days of special prayers and services of mourning and remembrance. All members in our group were not Catholic, but we wanted to express our solidarity in joining with the suffering of our host community. We were surprised that we received mixed responses from members of the community. While most were gracious and appreciative, others resentfully viewed our involvement as intrusive and unnecessary. As a result, we decided to return early to the central urban volunteer hub in Santiago to remove ourselves from the controversy and allow space for the community to heal. After a few days, we were able to return to our host families and proceed with the remainder of the program.

My experience highlights the delicate and necessary intersection of spirituality and healthcare, especially within the context of international and global health service work. Regardless of our own spirituality or convictions, as Americans, we come to these encounters unable to separate ourselves from our power and privilege. We cannot be effective healthcare providers unless we are willing to be vulnerable and engage with the spirituality and culture of those whom we serve. There were those in our group who were not Catholic or religious and therefore felt uncomfortable participating in the religious practices of the community, either due to a lack of familiarity or contradictions with their personal beliefs. As a Catholic myself, I was able to serve as a bridge for our group and to interpret the significance of the spiritual experience, but I still found it necessary to rely on the guidance and direction of the local community rather than assume my own practice or understanding of faith would be congruent with their experience and expectations. In our willingness to remove ourselves entirely, we were able to demonstrate humility and respect for the needs of the community. Rather than insist on proceeding with our planned work, we were able to pivot and serve with compassion while affirming the dignity of the community.

My experience in the Dominican Republic demonstrates the values of encounter and care for the whole person and has informed my personal mission as a pharmacist to provide spiritually inclusive care. I strive to use reflection and discernment to look into myself before encountering others. In this way, I can advocate for justice and demonstrate solidarity with the poor and marginalized through my work as a pharmacist in primary care at a community health center that focuses on migrant and seasonal farm workers and others with barriers to accessing care.

If I were asked to advise individuals who want to incorporate more spiritual care into their practice as a pharmacy professional, I would say that it is necessary to recognize the spiritual elements of a person as integral to their health regardless of our own practice or understanding of a particular faith tradition. Important skills include active listening, cultural humility, empathy, and a willingness to be present and adaptable. Genuine encounter and care for others must begin with a reflective understanding of our own spirituality and then shift the emphasis to the other person's lived experience. Pharmacists seeking to incorporate more spiritual care into their practice should demonstrate a respect for diverse belief systems and seek opportunities for cross-cultural experiences as well as collaborate with chaplains or other spiritual care providers. Our role as healthcare providers is not to proselytize or preach but to understand and appreciate how spirituality influences the health and medication outcomes of our patients.

Reference

1. Pope Francis. *Fratelli tutti: On fraternity and social friendship*. Vatican City, Vatican: Libreria Editrice Vaticana; 2020. Para 50.

A Pharmacist's Spiritual Journey While Working on American Indian Reservations

Kathryn Rose Thorsness Schultz
BS Pharm, PharmD, MPH, FASHP, FMSHP

"*Oki!*" means "greetings" in the Blackfoot language, and "*Boozhoo!*" is the Ojibwe way of saying "hello."

I became interested in doing contract work for the Indian Health Service (IHS) several years ago through a contact with a recruiter. The mission of the IHS is "to raise the physical, mental, social, and spiritual health of American Indians (AI) and Alaska Natives (AN) to the highest level." The IHS is continually seeking pharmacists to serve on the nation's reservations, which provide healthcare to 574 federally recognized AI and AN tribes. About 2.8 million people are served by the IHS of the nation's estimated 3.7 million AI and AN people. In addition to other healthcare professionals, approximately 790 pharmacists provide care to these patients in both rural and urban hospitals, health centers, and village clinics. I am one of those pharmacists and have served patients at the Blackfeet Reservation in Browning, MT, the Cheyenne River Health Service in Eagle Butte, SD, and the Fort Peck Reservation in Poplar, MT.

The AI and AN populations face significant health disparities, with a life expectancy approximately 10.9 years shorter than that of the US general population, and disproportionately higher rates of hypertension, heart disease, diabetes, pulmonary diseases, chronic kidney disease, and cancer. Alcohol use disorder, substance use disorder, and violence contribute significantly to excess mortality in AI/AN populations, with intentional harm/suicide, assaults, and homicides occurring at higher rates than in the US general population.

I have learned that Native Americans represent many distinct tribes, each with its own unique cultural and spiritual practices. This is unlike my experience in the Catholic Church where the worship service is very similar in Wisconsin, where I was raised, and in Belfast, Northern Ireland, where I visit on vacation. The order of the Mass, the prayers, and even hymns are similar, although individual Catholic parishes may have services in different languages, such as Latin, Spanish, or Vietnamese.

As examples of the diversity among the AI and AN communities where I have served, the Lac Courte Oreilles Band of Ojibwe, located near my hometown, is

DOI: 10.37573/9781585287727.024

one of six federally recognized bands of Ojibwe people in Wisconsin. Minnesota is home to 11 federally recognized tribes in both rural and urban areas. My first IHS position was in Browning, MT, home to the Blackfeet Indian, whose tribal members primarily belong to the Piegan Blackfeet band of the Blackfoot Confederacy, which spans both the United States and Canada. The Cheyenne River Sioux Tribe Reservation in SD is home to four of the traditional seven bands of the Lakota Nation: Mnicoujou (Plants by the Water); Itazipco (Sans Arc); Sihasaspa (Black Foot); and Oohenumpa (Two Kettles). Fort Peck, MT, is home to the Assiniboine and Sioux tribes.

Many Native Americans follow Christian beliefs. They may be Catholic, Baptist, or, like a patient I saw recently, Episcopalian. Many others follow indigenous Native American healing practices. Ceremonies to celebrate the seasons or giving thanks to the Creator and living in harmony with the earth have been traditional practices for thousands of years. Native American healing ceremonies typically include Christian symbolism and icons. Indigenous healers, commonly referred to as Medicine Men or Women, may attend the patient to pray with a sick person and their family.

The Cheyenne River Health System facility has a Spiritual Room for family members or others to gather, offer prayers, smudge or burn sage, or perform other acts that integrate traditional healing practices with conventional, allopathic medicine.

The patient in my story had a severe adverse reaction to a medication she had received. Her provider wanted to try another drug in the same class in the hope that it would be effective and tolerated and not cause a reaction. The patient told me that she was worried about this new medication and was afraid that she might die if she took it. She lived alone in a sparsely populated area of the reservation. This is not unusual. Reservations may be very large; many of the patients whom I have met must travel long distances to access healthcare. She shared with me that she was praying that she would be ok. I counseled her on the medication and gave her specific symptoms that she should watch for if the new medication caused a similar reaction. We talked about a plan where she might stay with her sister when starting the new medication, so she would have family supporting her, and she would be nearer to healthcare services. As our counseling session was ending, I saw that she was wearing a crucifix and asked her if she wanted me to pray with her. We said a brief prayer together.

After we prayed, she told me that she had gone on a "Spiritual Walk" to pray over her health. In a "Spiritual Walk," people pray as they walk a path that often leads to a higher ground or summit. Upon reaching the summit, she left a prayer tie with tobacco tied inside as an offering. A prayer tie may just be a bit of cloth in colors, such as red (representing strength and courage), white (peace or heaven), yellow (the sun or the dawn), blue (wisdom, the sky, water), or other colors with significant meanings. Tobacco is often tied inside to signify its special relationship with the Creator. The smoke from burning tobacco is believed to carry prayers and intentions to the Creator, with the tobacco itself holding the energy of the person offering it. I wished her well and thanked her for sharing her story. I was left with a feeling of gratitude for this patient who shared her personal story with me, and I hope that she will be more trusting of her healthcare providers, because I took time to listen to her health and spiritual concerns.

My work, willingness to meet and accept all people where they are, and an innate curiosity about others have given me an opportunity to learn about Native American practices and languages from coworkers and patients. I've gained a deeper appreciation of the importance of understanding how various tribes and their unique cultures incorporate their spiritual beliefs into their healthcare. The people with whom I have worked over the past several years have been gracious in teaching me about their cultures, languages, communities, the ubiquitous "Rez Dogs," and where to get the best Indian tacos. I have learned that cultural awareness, humility, and respect for all people I encounter will leave my patients, my coworkers, and me better because of our shared experiences.

Serving on several Native American reservations, I have discovered a lot of interesting facts about various Native American tribes and have come to discover a deeper personal faith in myself. The intersection of my own faith and that of my patients—be it Christian or Native Spirituality—has been a fascinating journey of growth for me. The interactions I've had with my patients in the IHS have deepened my understanding of different Native American cultural and religious beliefs and practices. I believe that I can provide better care for all patients if I take the time to listen to everyone I work with and care for, as well as learn about them as individuals, rather than make assumptions that their beliefs are all the same and identical to mine.

Miigwech ("Thank you" in Ashinaabewomin Ojibwe) to friends and coworkers and *Gazaagi'in* ("I love you" in Ojibwe) to my family for their support in this extraordinary journey.

Religious Education Meets Real-World Practice

Kathryn Schwaller
PharmD, MS

My life has largely been shaped by the influence of my faith. I grew up in a small, Protestant Christian town and attended a public high school where the influence of the church had significant impact. In college, I chose a similar path, enrolling in private, Christian liberal arts schools and then graduating from a Christian university with my Doctor of Pharmacy (PharmD) degree. In my first year of pharmacy school, I was honored to help select our class verse, 1 Peter 4:10, *"Each of you should use whatever gift you have received to serve others, as faithful stewards of God's grace in its various forms"* (New International Version [NIV]). This verse formed the foundation of our classwork as we were taught to love others, including the importance of how to talk to our patients about their spiritual health. My PharmD program emphasized that the spiritual health of our patients is a crucial part of caring for the whole person.

Within the four walls of pharmacy school, the concept seemed so simple: love others, ask permission to share the Gospel, and offer to pray with patients if they were interested. Practicing this presented challenges as we were assigned to advanced pharmacy practice experience (APPE) rotations at nonreligious hospitals. In our student discussion groups, we had the opportunity to process the implications of not having those conversations and how we might interact with our patients differently. However, after I completed school, I moved into residency training and realized that it wasn't always as easy to discuss spiritual health and engage in faith-based conversations with my mentors and co-workers. As I contemplated my future career path following my fourth year of pharmacy school, my faith, my husband's faith, and the prayers of many others all played a significant role in where I practice today. My path led me to a large children's medical center, which was established as a faith-based organization but currently is unaffiliated with any particular faith. I chose to pursue advanced training as a Health-System Pharmacy Administration and Leadership (HSPAL) resident, which involved a year of patient care training followed by a year primarily in an administrative role with some additional clinical experiences. My first year was mentally, emotionally, and spiritually challenging as I went from an environment where it was easy to discuss faith to real-world practice where conversations about spiritual health were few and far between. I had not anticipated the personal difficulties in shifting from a faith-based educational curriculum to a work setting where spirituality was not emphasized.

DOI: 10.37573/9781585287727.025

I realized that part of the challenge that I faced was learning how to carve out intentional time for my own spiritual nourishment and growth, so I could have meaningful faith-based conversations with others. Up to that point, my educational journey had included built-in time to nurture my faith, but the world outside those settings didn't offer the same structure. I had to proactively seek a church and community to support my faith development. Without this support, I had nothing to guide my faith nor encourage me to share my faith with my patients. In the early months of my residency, several of my patients passed away, and I found myself wrestling with the losses. At the hospital, the pharmacy was in the basement, and I saw family members passing the pharmacy on their way to the morgue as they faced their unfathomable loss. I found myself silently praying as I walked the hallways throughout the day. Initially, I prayed for my patients to live, but over time, I added prayers to ask God to grant peace to our families and care providers as we navigated difficult circumstances and the reality of death. This personal revelation put my training in a new light. Not only is the spiritual health of our patients important, but so is the spiritual health of their families and our staff.

In my second year of residency, I got to experience this in a different way when I was in conversation with my pharmacy team members. One of my pharmacy technicians told me that she prays over her medication deliveries. Other pharmacists and I have started having faith-based conversations about how our faith can drive our purpose as we answer the invitation to use our special gifts. I recall a conversation with a former employee who, after reviewing my resume, asked me about my education in faith-based schools. This encounter reminded me of a lecture in pharmacy school that emphasized the power of asking people questions about their faith to open doors to transformative conversations. The principles of caring for our patients and supporting our teams resonate regardless of the specific area of pharmacy where we practice.

Ironically, my skills for discussing spiritual health manifested themselves in a new way. Recently, my husband shared that he was distressed about one of his patients who was struggling after losing his wife. He asked for my advice on how to care for this patient, beyond dispensing and counseling the patient on his medications. I suggested that my husband pray for his patient privately and ask the patient if they could pray together. As their encounter unfolded, the patient expressed his own faith, and my husband asked his permission for our small group from church to pray for this individual as well. The next time my husband saw his patient, he shared that both of us and our small group at church had been praying for him. The patient expressed his thankfulness for the prayers.

My transition to real-world practice has taught me that developing your own faith and the skills to discuss spiritual health with others is incredibly important in providing whole-person care. Intentionally building time in my own schedule to invest in my faith opened my mind to see opportunities where I felt like God might be calling me to share my faith with others, whether that was with patients or colleagues who would then feel empowered to share their faith. I never know when opportunities might arise to discuss spirituality in the workplace, but I am glad that I received an education that prepared me for those moments. My advice to others wanting to incorporate spiritual care into their practice is to not suppress their faith, but instead to live it out in the day to day and not be afraid to share when the right opportunity presents itself.

Role of Prayer in Managing Patients with HIV/AIDS

Gary H. Smith
PharmD, FASHP, FCCP, FAPhA

When I was a faculty member at a school of pharmacy, my clinical position was at the infectious diseases clinic of the university medical center. My role was primarily receiving referrals to provide medication management for patients with human immunodeficiency virus (HIV)/autoimmune deficiency syndrome (AIDS) and other chronic diseases. The demographics of the clinic's patient population were primarily African American from the inner city. Most of the population acquired HIV infection from injection drug use with sexual transmission a distant second.

I am Christian and a member of a conservative Lutheran Church. For most of my role as a practitioner, I have carried out the practice of praying for or with each patient under my care. My usual approach would be to ask the patient if they would like me to pray for them, which usually took place at the end of the visit. I would inform the patient that I was a Christian and had observed that prayer often helped with the healing process. It was rare that anyone declined. In fact, most patients were surprised when I asked; I believe that it improved our relationship going forward. I would continue to pray for each patient daily if I was assisting with their care.

One of my patients was a 40-year-old African American woman who acquired HIV/AIDS through sexual intercourse with an HIV-positive male about 10 years before she was referred to my care. She was a single mother with two daughters, one of whom was also positive for HIV/AIDS acquired from her mother during pregnancy. Her older daughter was born prior to her infection with HIV. The patient was referred to me by her Nurse Practitioner (NP) for medication management and improvement in her compliance with her HIV medication regimen, but she was also being treated for hypertension and with an antibiotic to prevent another episode of pneumonia. She had been on multiple antiretroviral regimens due to resistance to several antiretroviral agents, which was most likely due to her lack of adherence to the prescribed regimen. Her viral level at this time was about 1,200 cells/mL (normal is an undetectable level). I consulted with the NP about her current medications, and she suggested that I review all the patient's medications, including her HIV medications, with the goal of simplifying them as much as possible. I suggested that due to noncompliance, I would monitor the patient's medication response initially on a weekly basis. We decided that the NP would give

DOI: 10.37573/9781585287727.026

her new prescriptions on her next visit and tell her to bring all her medications with her when she saw me at the next follow-up appointment.

My goals at our first visit were to introduce myself and to help her fill her pill boxes for 1 week. I discussed with her the importance of taking her medications each day as prescribed. We considered which times during the day would be the easiest for her to remember to take her medications. She promised to take all her medications and to work hard to do better than she had in the past. We reviewed possible side effects, and I emphasized that if she found them unmanageable to call me as I might be able to provide help to relieve the effects. As my usual close of a visit, I told her that I was a Christian and asked her if she would like me to pray for her. She said that she would welcome prayer and thanked me for offering it. I assured her that I would pray for her every day as long as she was under my care and would call her once a week. For the first month, we met weekly. Our visits consisted of discussing whether she had been taking her medications as prescribed, assessing her viral load, and giving her positive support on how well she was doing. Her adherence was good, only missing 1 day each week during the first 2 weeks and missing no medications in the last 2 weeks of the first month. She was tolerating the medications well and was pleased with her progress. The viral load steadily decreased, down to 600 cells/mL after the first month and eventually became undetectable.

We prayed together at the end of each visit for continued good progress and to keep a positive attitude. After 4 weeks, we decided to change our appointments to every 2 weeks for the next month and, if all went well, every month for the next 4 months. She informed me that she had been praying daily and thought that the prayers were most likely the reason she was doing so well. She had not had anyone pray for her health before nor had she thought of doing it herself. I felt we had developed an excellent relationship, because she never missed an appointment and always had a positive attitude. I had made notes to that effect in her medical record. The NP saw the patient every 6 months and reviewed my notes at each visit. The NP said that she noticed a huge change in the patient's attitude after she started seeing me. The NP admitted that at one point she thought the patient would die from AIDS, but the patient's happiness and desire to comply with her treatment regimen after our visits proved to be a bright spot that could change the patient's health journey to recovery.

In summary, I believe that praying for my patients makes a difference in their outcome. This patient thought it made a big difference and voiced that she wished that someone had prayed for her sooner.

This story conveys what I hope my students will understand. My clinical site served as an ambulatory care rotation for fourth-year pharmacy students. After being with me for a few weeks and observing my interaction with the patients, I usually allowed the student to meet with them alone and report their assessment back to me. I would then meet with the patient briefly to see if they had any questions and to pray. One student had met with the above patient alone and told me afterwards that she had told him I had saved her life. I had never had a patient say anything like that before.

After 4 years at the clinic, I took a new position. The medical director of the clinic said she was sorry to see me go and told me that I had made a big impact on the care of my patients. I responded to her that it was due to the power of prayer, and she agreed.

I didn't always pray for my patients, but the older I got the more comfortable I felt incorporating spirituality into my practice. It created a bond that allowed the patient to trust me, and it often proved positive in their therapeutic outcomes. I have incorporated prayer in my own life, including praying for my students, and it has provided me with guidance in my career. In many of my professional positions, I felt underqualified for the position, but my prayers helped me to remain humble, knowing that my skills and talents were needed to care for my patients.

Celebrating Life After a Close Encounter with Death

Claudia N. Swenson
PharmD, FASHP

I am a pharmacist who has been trained to provide direct patient care in both inpatient and outpatient settings and served as a clinical coordinator at two health systems. I practiced in these settings for more than 40 years, primarily in the Pacific Northwest, and "retired" almost 10 years ago. However, there is still a strong need for my services, and I have continued to practice part-time, in mainly ambulatory settings. Through a local seniors' organization that I founded, I provide both spiritual and medical support to patients in my community. My spirituality is one that I share with my husband, also a pharmacist, and other family members. I am sharing one example where I have provided pharmacist care and spiritual support to a patient and the benefit that we both have gained from our experiences together.

During the final year of his wife's life, a local gentleman sought support from the care organization for seniors where I volunteer. The organization is a local nonprofit that helps seniors remain in their homes for as long as is safely possible. It provides support through one-on-one visits with a trained care volunteer. Our most common visits are around friendship and reducing social isolation. The initial assessment is comprehensive: demographics, physical ability, chronic conditions, family/friend/church or other spiritual support, and social determinants of health. As the organization's manager and board president and a clinical pharmacist, I provide support for two to three clients with complex medical issues.

My client and his wife were very active in their community, developing strong bonds with several local families, and participated in supporting children in schools through a grandparent's program. My client's wife had broken her back in an accident 20 years prior while helping their son build a home. Their children both lived 6 hours away. My client and his wife communicated with their son and daughter mainly by telephone, email, and text messaging. Despite being wheelchair-bound, my client's wife was very active in her nondenominational Christian church, especially in Bible studies and serving as a mentor to many.

In the last 2 years of her life, my client's wife required skilled nursing care in a larger community that was 45 miles away. Due to finances, he needed to ride the bus to visit her, and he faithfully visited her three times each week until she passed. Our senior care organization provided twice-monthly transportation and lunch to support him during this challenging time, along with friendly visits to encourage him personally. Our conversations often centered around God's strength and grace

DOI: 10.37573/9781585287727.027

for his journey. His wife developed dementia during the final 6 months of life, adding challenges in honoring and loving her until the end.

At 83 years of age, my client continued to live in their small home, taking care of both inside and outside tasks. One snowy day after Christmas 2022, he chose to shovel snow, felt chest discomfort, and came inside to lie down. He chose to call 911. The emergency medical service (EMS) unit was 2 blocks away and quickly responded. As the emergency medical technicians were loading him into the ambulance, his heart went into ventricular fibrillation. He was "shocked" back into normal rhythm and was intubated. Again, he experienced wide complex tachycardia requiring medication and cardioversion. He was transported to a hospital 50 miles away where he received care in the cardiac catheterization lab, which included a balloon pump and multiple medications to stabilize his blood pressure and circulation. During this time, messages about his condition went out to friends from Mexico to Alaska and prayers began pouring in. Along the way, a rumor of his "death" started to circulate, but it quickly corrected. He was extubated after 3 days and had an uneventful recovery; he was discharged home within a week.

Statistics show that $< 10\%$ of patients survive out-of-hospital cardiac arrest. His nurses called him the miracle patient. His physicians were amazed by his recovery. He strongly felt the support and was so thankful for the prayers of his church and community friends.

I now accompany him to all medical specialty appointments. He knows that I will listen carefully, provide clarification of issues, and help him to understand the benefits and risks of any regimen or testing (ie, antiarrhythmics, anticoagulation, blood pressure control, echocardiography). His internist, cardiologist, and anticoagulation provider have verbalized appreciation for the support that I provide during his appointments and follow-up care.

His trust in me is based on our mutual understanding of life's meaning and challenges and our trust in God. He recently wanted to explore the wisdom of having surgery for hernia repair now, while he is in good health, compared with waiting until it requires more urgent care. After careful discussion with his cardiology and internal medicine providers, he is comfortable with "watchful waiting."

My client continued to regain strength, walking both inside and outside. For safety, he uses a Medical Alert device, allows a neighbor to check on him if his window blinds aren't up in the early morning, and texts his daughter daily. He has returned to his hobby as a ham radio operator and to leading a Bible study group. The story of his ordeal and recovery is so compelling that he was invited to be the guest speaker at the local EMS annual banquet. He also continues to provide friendship and support to others. Through his own participation as a volunteer in the seniors' care program, he visits his best friend, who has pulmonary hypertension, twice a week. In addition to encouraging his friend mentally and emotionally, he does his pulmonary rehabilitation routines with him by using a stair master and treadmill. He has helped to start a Bible study in his friend's home.

This has been a growing experience for my client. He admits that his near-death experience has changed him emotionally as well as physically. He is more open to sharing his life's experiences with others and says, "Though I live alone, I never feel alone. I phone, email, and text friends. I also feel God's presence more with me now, and I pray more."

He continues to work hard to stay healthy, working out three times per week and walking in local stores. He has battled weight problems for years and diligently continues to keep his weight stable. He truly considers the last 2 years of living a "gift from God" and celebrates each day! His personal journey, facing life with determination, courage, and faith, and the courageous journeys of other seniors have been so enriching to my life. Their journeys help me, at age 78, to remain involved in pharmacy and several nonprofits in my community. By reaching out and helping others, we gain strength for our days and always receive back so much more than we give.

When Ripples Become Waves

Elva Angelique Van Devender
PhD, PharmD, BCPS, DPLA

I never planned to make waves on my first day of clinical rotations as a pharmacy student. My very first assignment was an intensive care unit (ICU) rotation at a prestigious 500-bed hospital with neurosurgery, cardiac, and medical ICUs that was over 2 hours away from my home. I had driven by the hospital earlier that morning so that I would know how to get there and where to park. I wanted to allow plenty of time to get my bearings before starting at 7 a.m. sharp. Critical care pharmacy was my favorite area of pharmacy. I enjoyed the pharmacology, the team-based environment, and the responsibility of caring for the sickest patients in the hospital. Working in the ICU requires nerves of steel and the ability to be a master of triage and an encyclopedia of clinical knowledge. I loved the fast-paced nature of it and the challenge of always having to be on your toes. Every day was different. Many of the ICU pharmacists at the hospital had storied careers where they practiced at the top of their license every day—playing an indispensable role during rounds, in consults, and participating in code blues (medical emergencies). Of all the medical emergencies that I attended in my career, one stands out for me, and it was the very first one on my first day.

The patient was 19 years old, and her mother was in the room when the patient coded. Things started happening quickly. My preceptor jumped into motion and started pulling the drugs out of the cart. The patient's room became a blur of blue scrubs and a whirl of organized commotion as each team member snapped into their specific roles within seconds. I knew immediately that there was nothing I could do for the patient that wasn't already being done by people far more experienced and capable than me, so my gaze fell on the only other person in the room who looked as wide-eyed and powerless as I did—the patient's mother. She was shaking as I located a chair for her to sit in and found some warm blankets to wrap around her. I introduced myself and knelt at her feet so that we would be roughly at eye level. I began explaining what each member of the team would be doing and what procedures would be performed, so she would not be so frantic about what was happening to her daughter. I offered her my hand, which she grabbed and held tightly. I told her, "I know this is overwhelming. I am here and will not leave you. God is here, and his servants are here to comfort and care for you and your daughter."

Normally I do not speak about my faith so openly, especially not at work. Maybe it was because the mother was wearing a cross. Maybe it was because I heard her cry out to Jesus. Maybe it was because when I looked down at our hands I

DOI: 10.37573/9781585287727.028

couldn't tell where hers left off and mine began. Talking about God at work (normally a taboo topic) just felt right to me in that moment. When I ran out of words to say, I put my arm around her and prayed with her. We recited Psalm 23 together. I didn't know what else to do. I felt ill-equipped to find soothing words in such an emotional and tumultuous setting.

The woman's daughter did not survive. In the aftermath of the code, her mother threw her arms around me, and I just held her while she sobbed. Someone from the team called the hospital chaplain for the mother (with her blessing). I was grateful the hospital had someone especially trained in comforting people who are grieving and have experienced loss. In our moments of grief, I do not believe it matters what respective belief system we come from. What matters is the kindness and compassion that we give to each other because of our shared humanity.

What mattered the most my first day on rotation was not my masterful knowledge of critical care guidelines and protocols. It was being present and my willingness to walk alongside someone in their grief. Typically, we don't train pharmacists or student pharmacists in spiritual care or how to serve others during stressful or emotional times. We assume that these matters are better left to someone else, perhaps a nurse or a chaplain who is more skilled in the art of support and who is involved more directly at the bedside with patients and family. Sadly, nurses are busy and cannot possibly do it all, and not all hospitals have spiritual caregivers available on a moment's notice. Even at the large hospital where I was trained, the chaplain wasn't called until the medical emergency was over.

In the weeks following the event, several people stopped me in the hallways of the ICU to tell me that they remembered me from that day and how I had cared for the patient's mother. One of the more senior ICU nurses thanked me and told me that I made her remember "why [she] went into healthcare in the first place." I was surprised that anyone had noticed, as I felt my contributions in the room were trivial compared with the actions of the skilled doctors, nurses, and my preceptor who provided direct patient care that day. My actions seemed small, but they had a ripple effect on everyone around me. My ICU preceptor told me years later that he never viewed a code the same after that one. He said, "After you did what you did, completely green, out of the gate, it made me see things differently. It made me reflect on the importance of what we do and what we sometimes fail to do. It also made me recognize all the helpers around me in my own life that I missed before." He told me that my actions strengthened his faith and purpose as a believer and as a pharmacist. The ripples from this experience also influenced my own professional career as a critical care and an emergency medicine pharmacist. Sometimes all I can offer patients is a kind smile, some water, and a warm blanket. Oftentimes, these things matter more to my patients than the medicine I am able to give them.

This experience taught me one of the greatest lessons of my professional practice: every action has a ripple effect. Even when we feel invisible (and pharmacy is often an invisible hand guiding medication usage in a hospital setting), actions matter. People matter. And waves that cause impactful outcomes can arise from the smallest of ripples.

We are all shaped by our beliefs, and we bring these elements into our work whether we talk about them openly or not. The values that we hold are extremely important guiding principles in all the decisions that we make and the work that we do as pharmacists, even if we are not consciously aware of their influence. I am the person that I am because of what I believe about myself, my world, and my purpose in the world. My belief in the interconnectedness of humanity—that we are all connected to each other and what happens to one member affects us all. This common human bond helps me find meaning, purpose, and connection in my career as a pharmacist as well as in my personal relationships with others.

My Traveling Companion

Carly B. Warner
PharmD, BCPS, BCGP

Traveling is something that spirituality and careers have in common. Whether on a spiritual journey or a career path, we are all traveling. Intersections are pivotal junctions in our travels, busy places where a lot is happening, choices are made, and directions are set. What happens at the intersection of a spiritual journey and a career path? What choices are made? What direction is taken?

Born and raised in the Christian faith, I have been thankful to find that my spiritual journey has paired nicely with my career path. I prayerfully considered a career in pharmacy, seeking out mentors who shared my faith and my hopeful future career. Pharmacy school is where I found my first intersection. My pharmacy school was home to a chapter of Christian Pharmacists Fellowship International (CPFI), and I was thrilled to join and serve. Quickly, I realized that being a pharmacist could deepen my faith. I have enjoyed exploring different career opportunities in pharmacy, including industry, community, hospital, residency, rehabilitation, organizational involvement, precepting, and research. My career path has had many more intersections than my spiritual journey, and at every turn different worlds collided. Consider the intersection of industry with its desks, meetings, tall office buildings, and community pharmacy with lines of patients, stacks of medication bottles, and ringing phones. Further along the path was the intersection of hospital with its verification queues, sterile compounding cleanrooms, dispensing machines, and residency training with a rush of codes, pharmacokinetic calculations, and patient counseling. So many different sights, sounds, and even patients in a variety of stages in their health journey.

Regardless of differences in my spiritual journey and career path, I realized in both that I was traveling. Sometimes I felt like I was traveling at the speed of light when I was enduring long hours in training. I looked toward the consistency and sturdiness that I had felt in my spiritual journey, and I came to understand that for my career path, I needed a traveling companion. What, like my faith, was always with me?

The answer is simple, so ingrained in our routines that it is easy to overlook. It is my badge. It looks different from organization to organization, but it is always there with my name and usually a photo (hopefully a good one) of my smiling face. One small addition transformed my badge into an intersection of my spiritual journey and my career path. A simple silver cross pin, representing my Christian faith.

DOI: 10.37573/9781585287727.029

Many days my cross simply helps to start my days centered with a quick prayer as I clip on my badge. On tough days, it catches the light as I look into the mirror while washing my hands, telling me my work has meaning and to keep serving. More times and ways than I can count, my cross, my traveling companion, has been a connector. A coworker asks if we can pray together after the loss of a patient or a difficult patient encounter. An exhausted caregiver points and says, "that cross on your badge gives me hope." A patient stopping in for counseling notices my cross pin and asks about my faith, shares theirs, and asks how they can pray for me and for our pharmacy. Patients have brought me faith-based gifts, beautiful cross-stiches, and prayer cards. At times, I have noticed a patient wearing a cross or other religious symbol, and I pointed to mine as a great conversation starter and a way to build rapport. The connections have stretched from fleeting to enduring; yet they have all been meaningful and undoubtedly deepened my faith and made me a better pharmacist.

Beyond connection, the consistent presence of the cross on my badge has challenged me to find other ways my spirituality can impact my practice. Now, when assessing information about a patient before I visit with them, I look for chaplain notes. On rounds, my recommendations have gone beyond medications on multiple occasions to mention that a call to the chaplain might be beneficial or to provide a referral to a clinic with faith-based providers when I know that is important to the patient. I now consider the ways spirituality or religious practices impact my patients' approach to their health and their medications. I have learned about the diverse spiritualities of my coworkers. I have read and exchanged books on spirituality in healthcare with patients and colleagues. On days when I felt I could not answer one more phone call, question, or experience another negative encounter, my cross pin challenged me to push through and keep going with grace. My career path has twisted through many very different frontiers of pharmacy; yet my cross has remained a constant, comforting traveling companion in every practice site.

Thankfully, I have not encountered a negative reception to the cross on my badge. I have been asked quite directly "Why do you have a cross on your badge?" My answer is usually a version of "to share with others what makes me the best pharmacist I can be." Often this leads to an exchange where I learn something about the inquirer, but occasionally my answer has been met with a silent nod, shrug, or smile. More times than I care to admit, my actions have not lived up to the values of my faith. In those instances, my cross pin offers the first nudge to reflect on how I could improve in the future. I am thankful my experience so far confirms the spiritual aspects of healthcare and that most patients appreciate the dialogue.

Over the years, I have added other pins to my badge, such as my alma maters, years of service milestones, or Board of Pharmacy Specialties certifications. They too represent intersections and give me the chance to share stories or inspire others. I admit when I first added the cross to my badge, it was mostly for me. It was my traveling companion. The pin represented my certainty in the face of all the unknowns that have accompanied my various career paths. Although small, my cross pin has been a source of great strength and has led to openness, sharing, and connectedness with my patients and coworkers.

Caring for the whole person means recognizing that health and well-being extend beyond the physical body. As defined by each patient, spirituality can play a significant role in how individuals experience illness, healing, and care.

These self-reflection questions are designed to help you explore your own beliefs, values, and experiences related to spirituality and whole-person care as both a provider and a patient. There are no right or wrong answers—only an invitation to pause and go deeper to better understand how we give, receive, and understand our healthcare journeys.

Questions for Reflection for Both Providers and Patients

1. Are there any stories in this collection with which you personally identify? If so, can you determine why these stories resonated with you?

2. Were there any stories that particularly surprised you? If so, why?

3. What steps would you take to challenge yourself to step outside of the ease/comfort/convenience zone if you find yourself in situations like the narratives in this collection?

Questions for Reflection for Providers

1. Reflect on a time when you may have chosen to avoid discussing or addressing the spiritual needs of a patient. As you read through these narratives, would you choose differently if the situation presented itself again?

2. What are some ways in which you may create a more welcoming environment for patients to approach you about their spiritual needs?

DOI: 10.37573/9781585287727.BM

Questions for Reflection for Patients

1. Reflect on a time when you may have chosen to avoid discussing your spiritual needs with a healthcare provider. Can you identify the cause of your reluctance? If the situation occurs again, will you choose differently?

2. If prayer is a part of your spiritual life, would you be comfortable offering to pray for your provider at the conclusion of your visit?

Self-Examination Questions in Anticipation of a Healthcare Provider and Patient Visit

For Healthcare Providers:

Before the patient visit

1. What are my own beliefs and values about spirituality, and how might they influence my healthcare goals?

2. Am I comfortable discussing spiritual needs with patients? Why or why not?

3. Am I comfortable asking about spiritual needs with patients who may be of a different faith than myself or express that they are nonreligious or nonspiritual?

4. Have I made assumptions about this patient's spiritual or religious identity prior to the visit that should be clarified during the visit?

5. How can I create a safe, confidential, and respectful space for this encounter?

During the discussion

6. Am I actively listening to the patient without judgment or bias?

7. Am I allowing the patient to define what spirituality means for them?

8. Am I using open-ended, inclusive language and questions that demonstrate respect for the patient's religion or spirituality even if it is different from my own?

9. Am I careful to distinguish between spiritual care and proselytizing?

After the patient visit

10. Did I understand the patient's spiritual concerns or needs clearly and document them, so they are communicated clearly to other members of the healthcare team?

11. What was the patient's response? Did they seem supported and heard, or did they perceive that their needs were being dismissed?

12. Is there anything that I would choose to do differently when I see the patient the next time to better support their spiritual well-being?

13. Did I ask the patient if they would like to speak with a chaplain or other spiritual care provider for additional support?

For Patients:

Before your next visit with a healthcare provider

1. What does spirituality mean to me, and how does it impact my health or healing?

2. Am I comfortable discussing my spiritual beliefs with my healthcare provider?

3. Are there specific spiritual practices or rituals that I want respected during my care?

4. What am I hoping to gain from a conversation with my healthcare provider about my spiritual needs?

During the visit

5. Am I being honest and clear about my needs or concerns?

6. Do I feel safe and respected in this conversation?

7. Am I comfortable asking for a chaplain, spiritual advisor, or someone else to support me?

After the visit

8. Do I feel like my provider listened to and respected my beliefs?

9. Was anything left unsaid that I might want to bring up later?

10. What else do I need—spiritually or emotionally—to feel more supported in my care?